YOU GOT THIS

WHEN IN DOUBT   JUST REMEMBER

THIS JOURNAL IS DEDICATED TO YOU. TO WHO YOU ARE IN THE PRESENT — TO THE GOALS AND DREAMS YOU ASPIRE TO ACHIEVE. TO YOUR SUCCESSES & FAILURES OF WHICH YOU WILL GROW AND EVOLVE. TO YOUR OPEN MIND, HEART, & SOUL. HAVE FUN, DREAM BIG, WORK HARD, AND BELIEVE IN YOU.

table of contents

❧ organization
CONTACTS
CALENDAR

❧ Habits
SELF-CARE
FITNESS TRACKER
NUTRITION & HEALTH

❧ Affirmations & Aspirations
INTENTIONS
GOALS
WORLD MAP & TRAVEL
JOURNALING
WONDER WOMEN

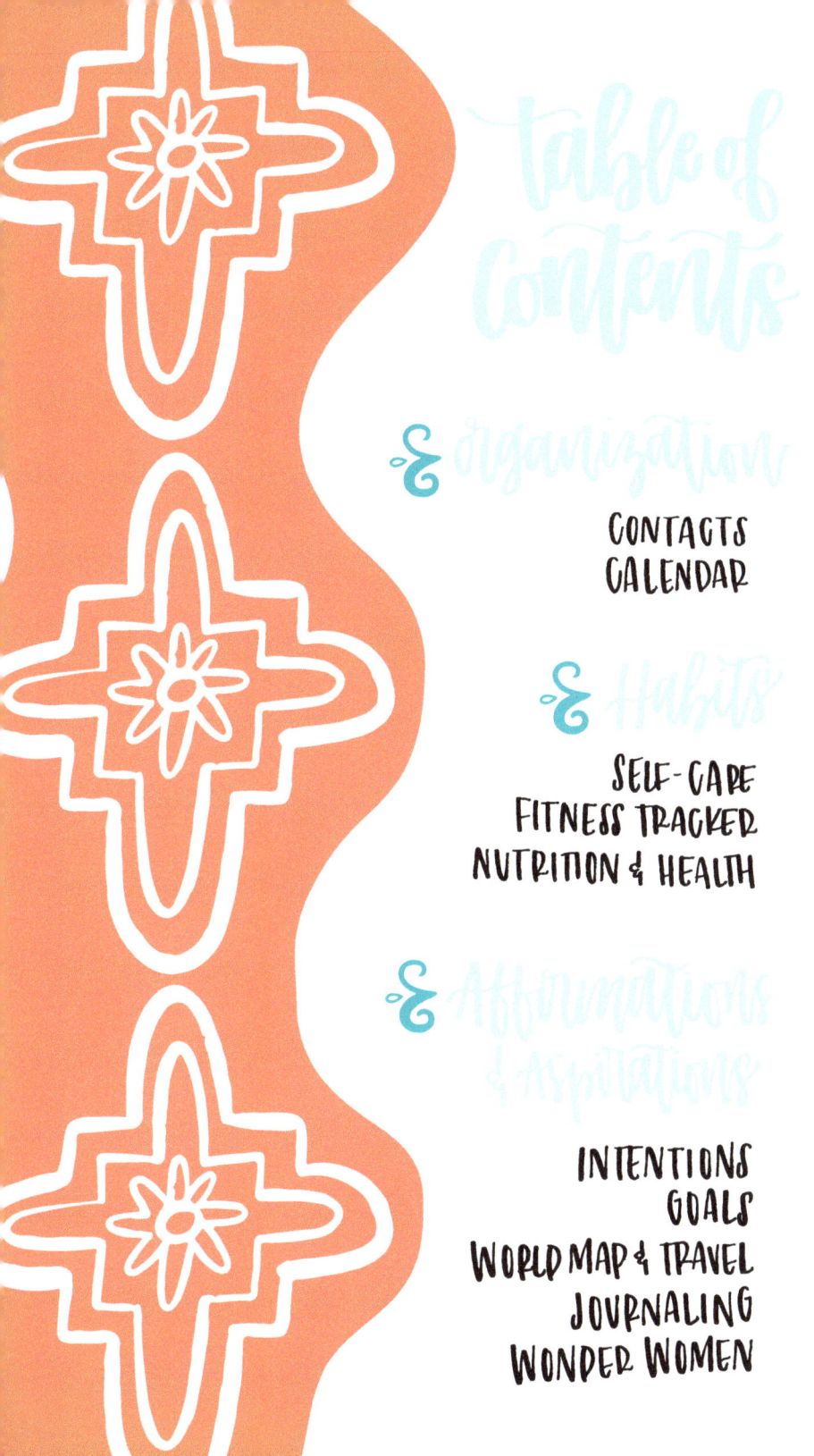

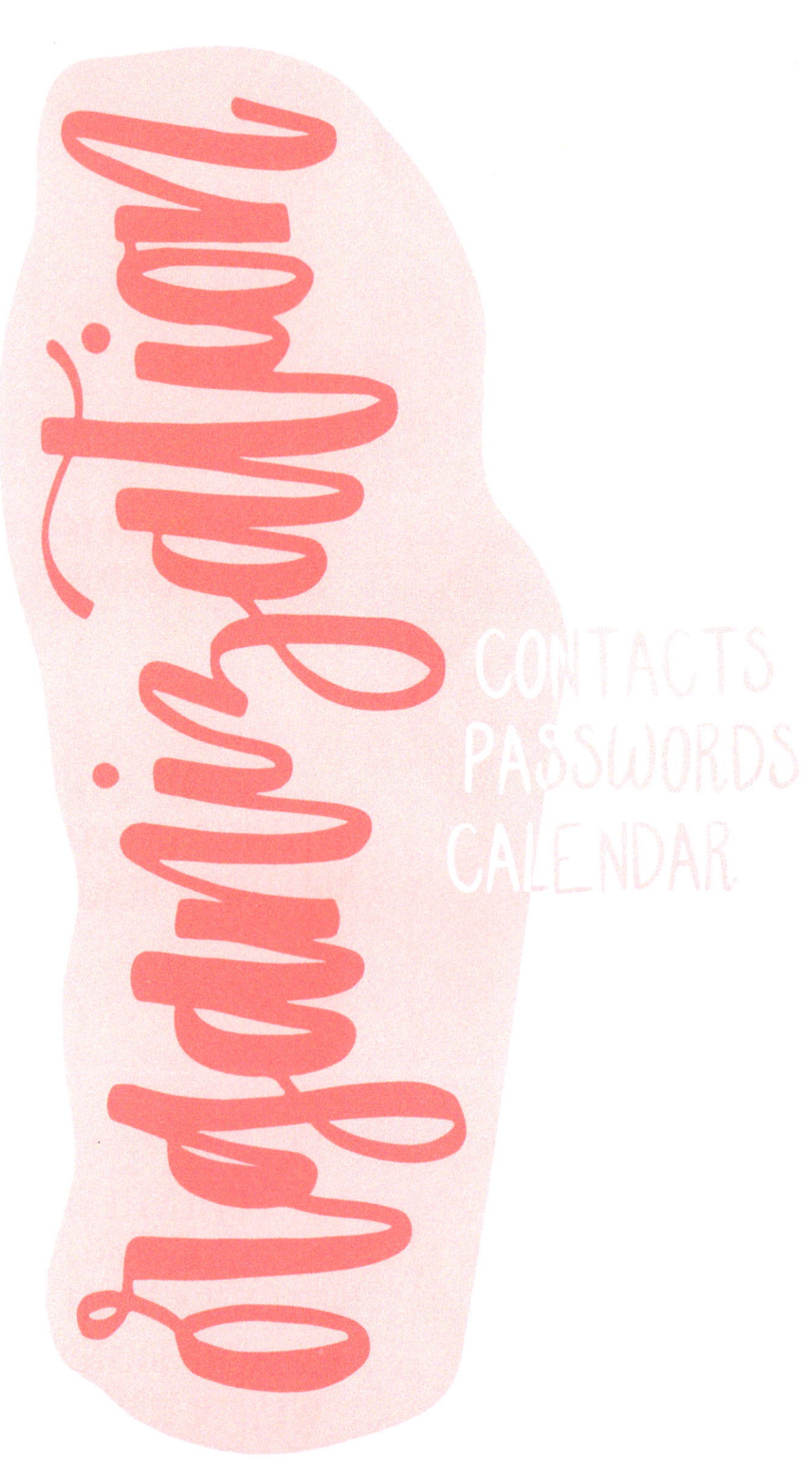

CONTACTS

name: _____
email: _____
phone #: _____
address: _____

name: _____
email: _____
phone #: _____
address: _____

name: _____
email: _____
phone #: _____
address: _____

name: _____
email: _____
phone #: _____
address: _____

name: _____
email: _____
phone #: _____
address: _____

name: _____
email: _____
phone #: _____
address: _____

IMPORTANT INFORMATION

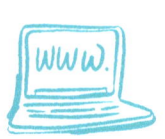   

WEBSITE	USERNAME	PASSWORD	EMAIL

calendar

A 12 month space to record events, birthdays, notes to self, and all that your heart desires!

Birthdays, events, notes,

January

1
2
3
4
5
6
7
8
9
10
11
12
13
14
15

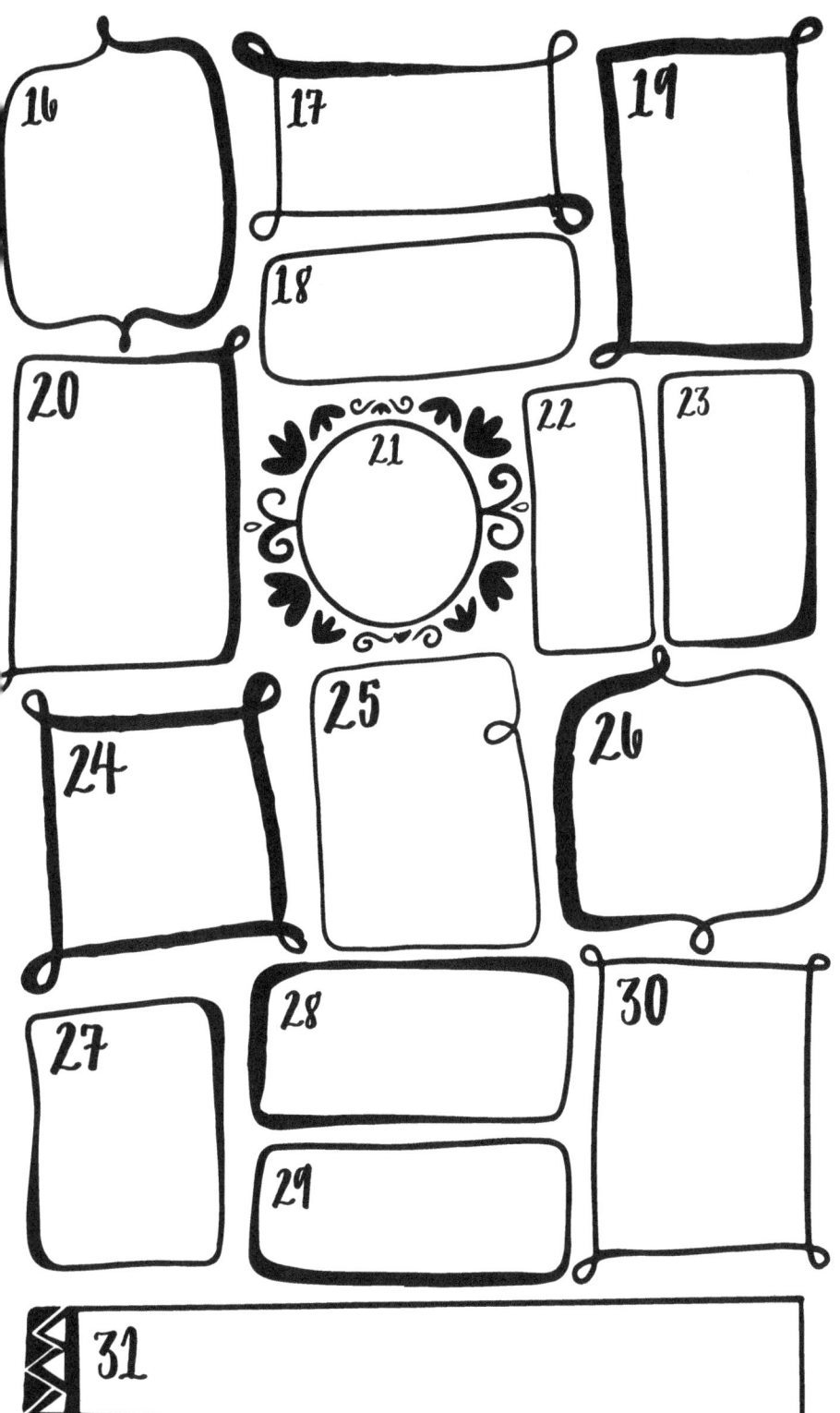

Birthdays, events, notes,

February

1
2
3
4
5
6
7
8
9
10
11
12
13
14
15

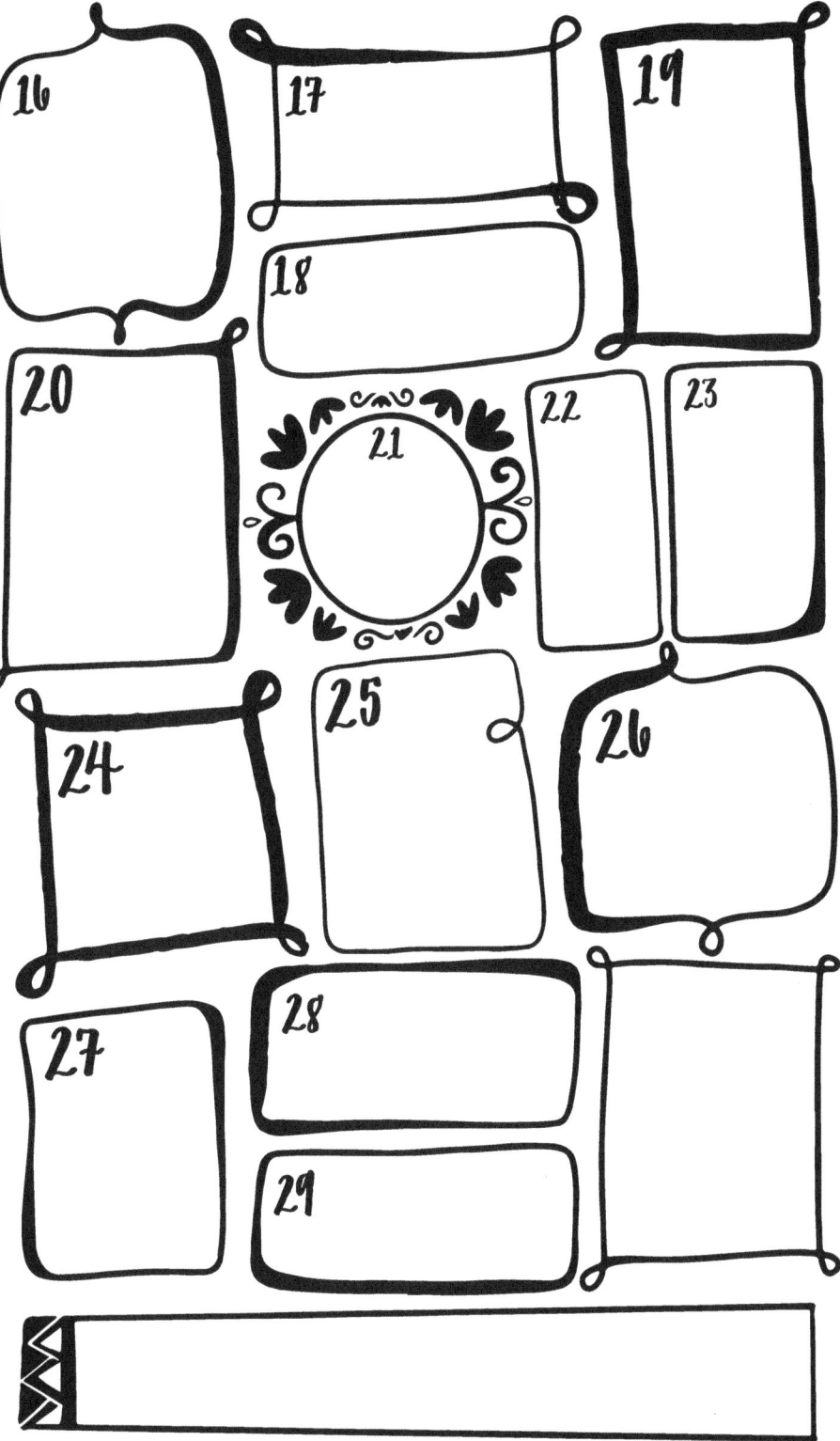

Birthdays, events, notes,

march

1
2
3
4
5
6
7
8
9
10
11
12
13
14
15

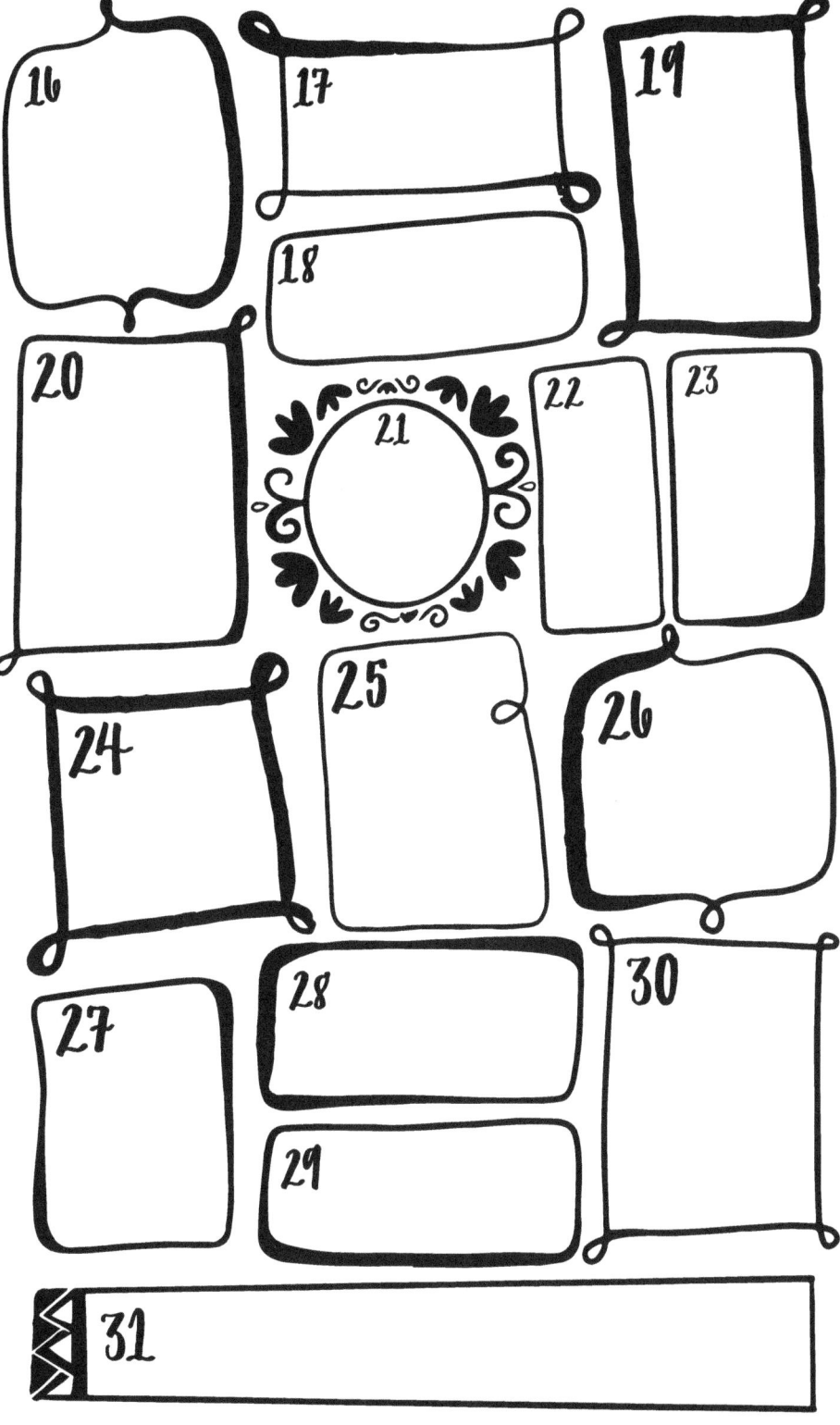

Birthdays, events, notes,

April

1
2
3
4
5
6
7
8
9
10
11
12
13
14
15

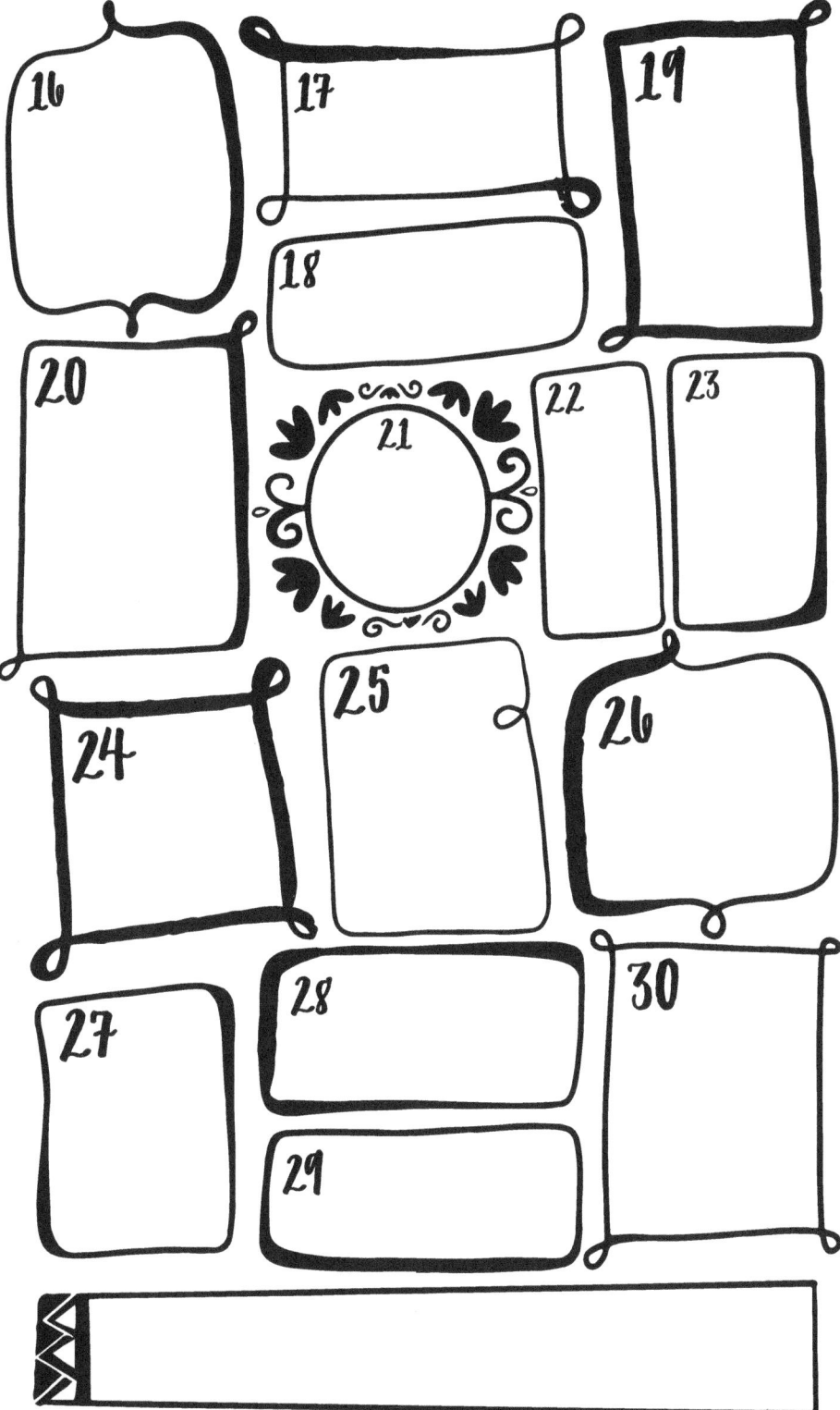

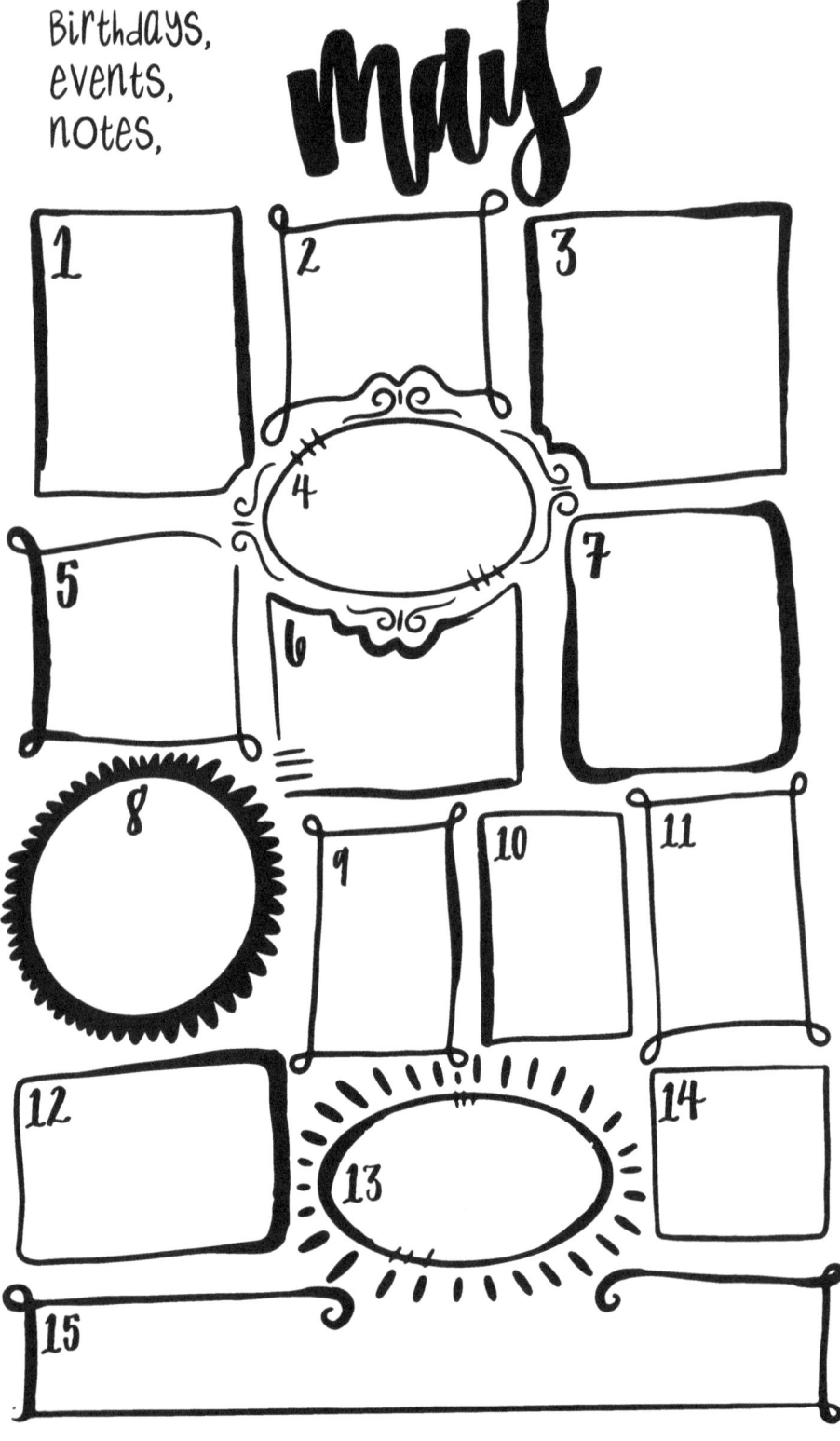

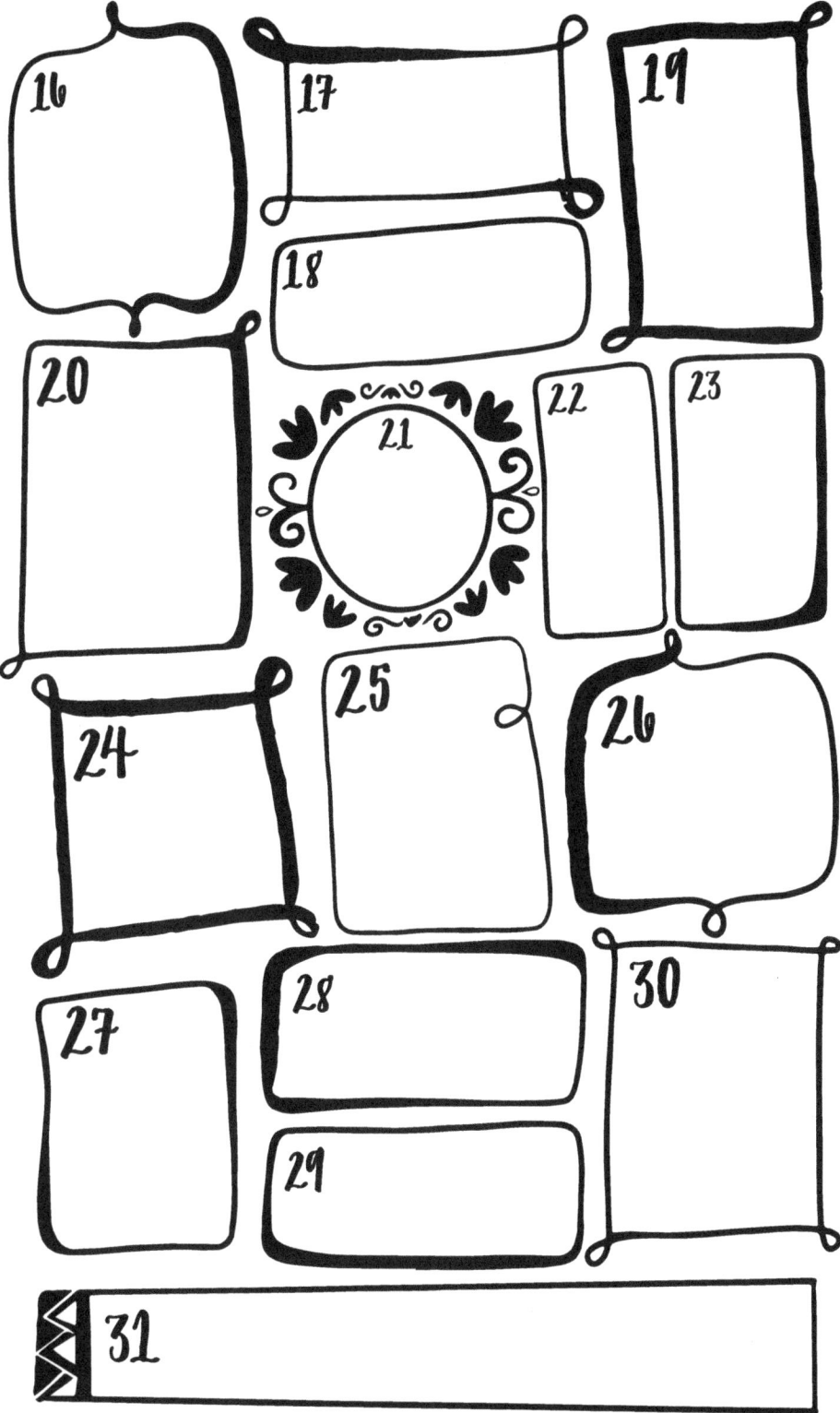

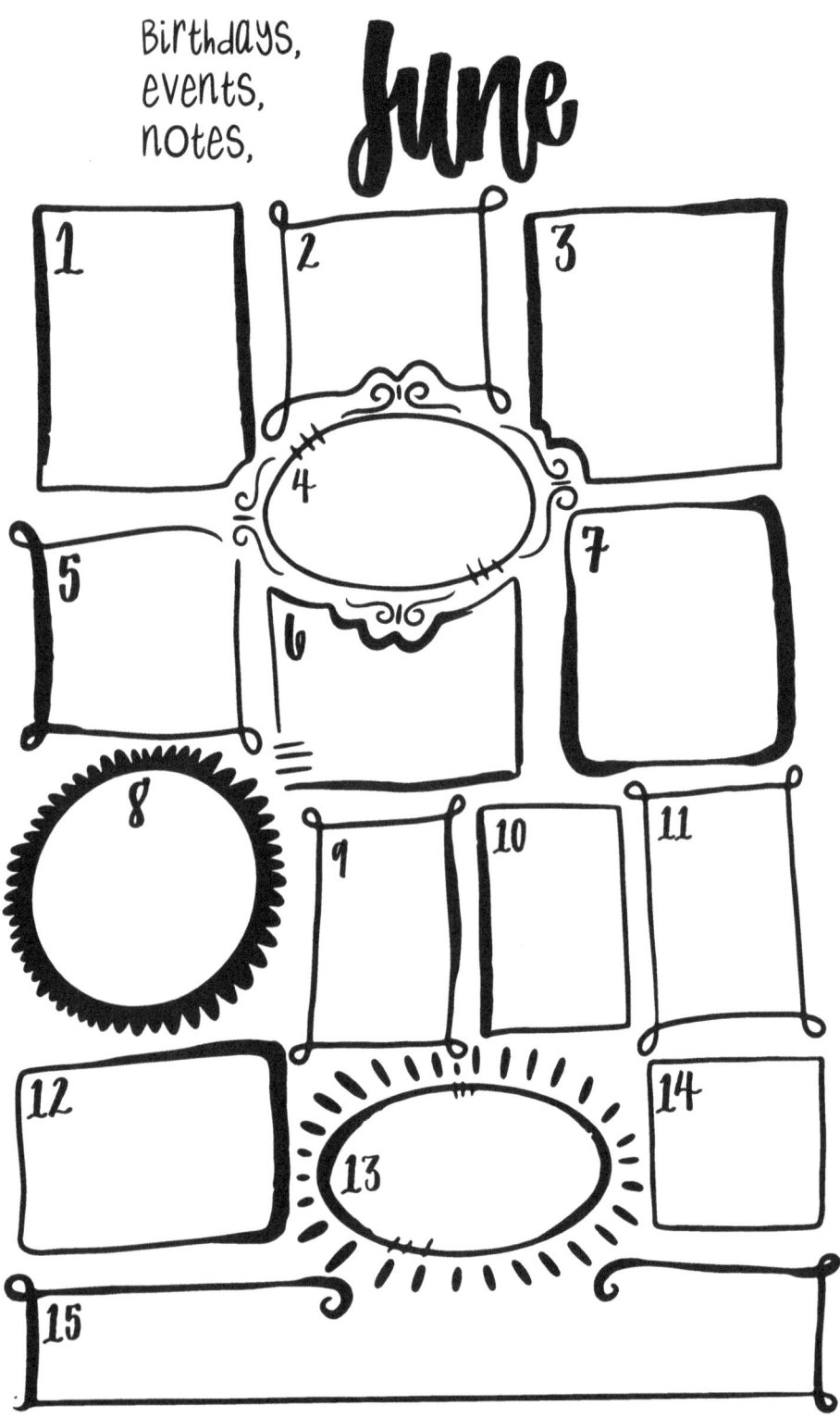

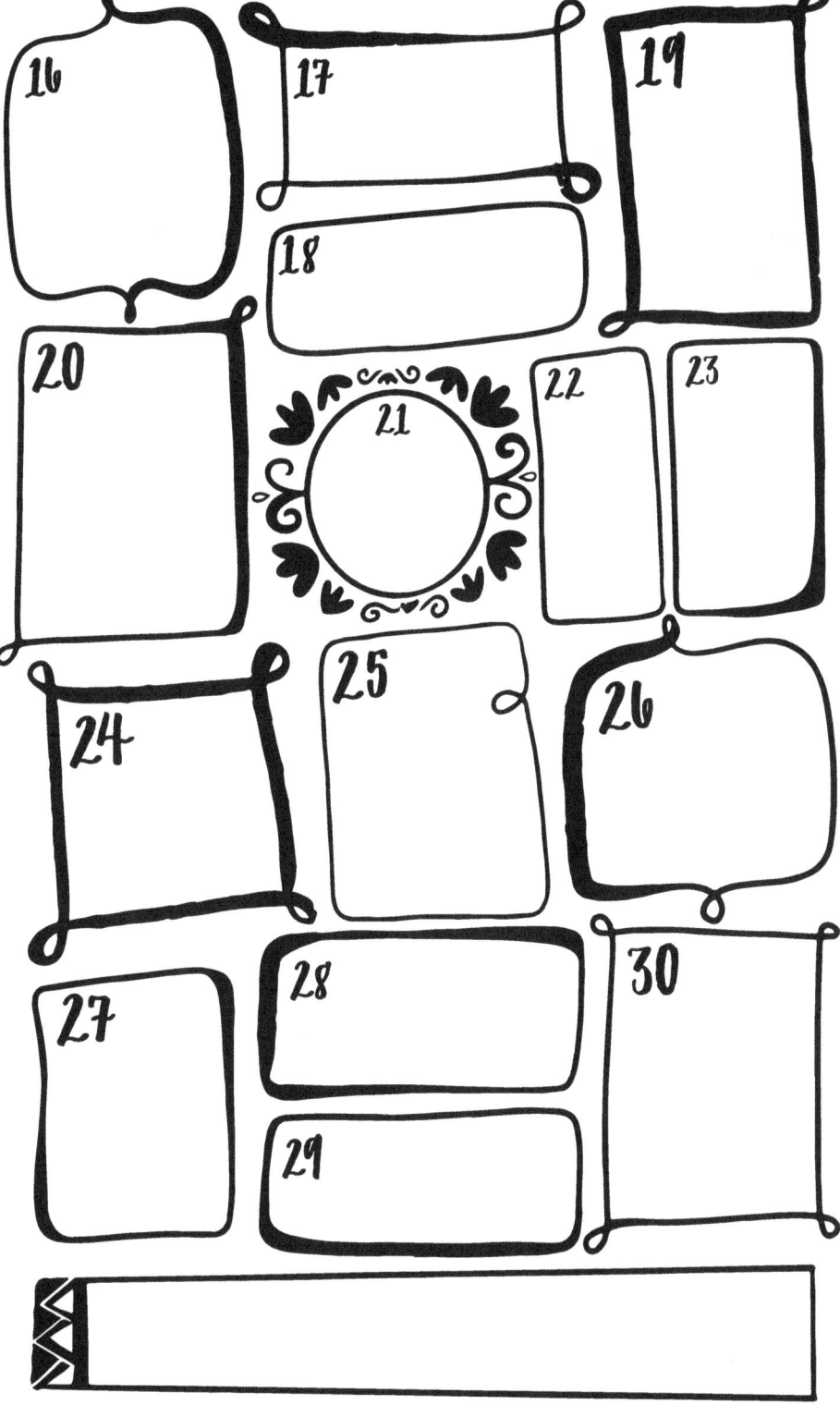

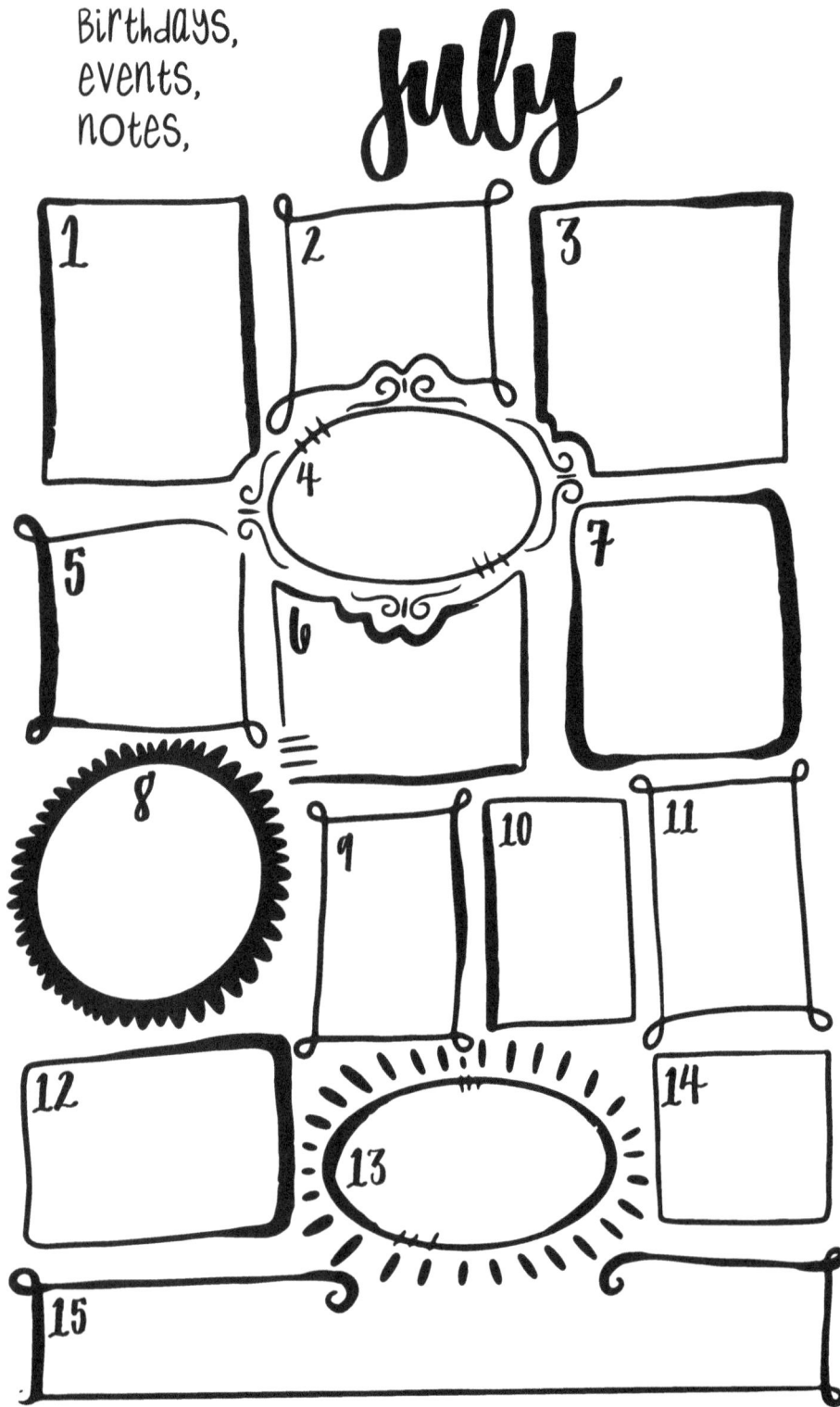

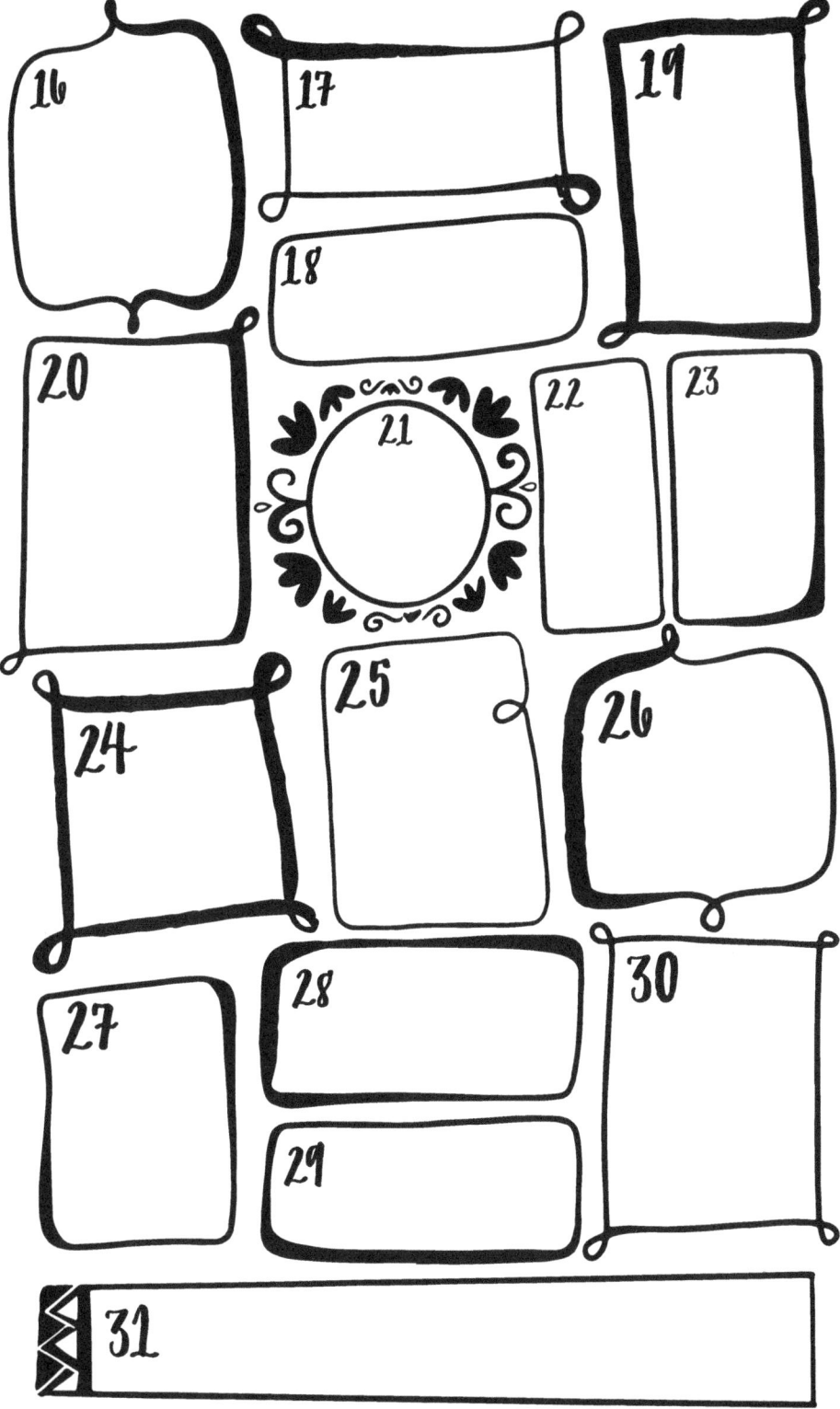

Birthdays, events, notes,

August

1
2
3
4
5
6
7
8
9
10
11
12
13
14
15

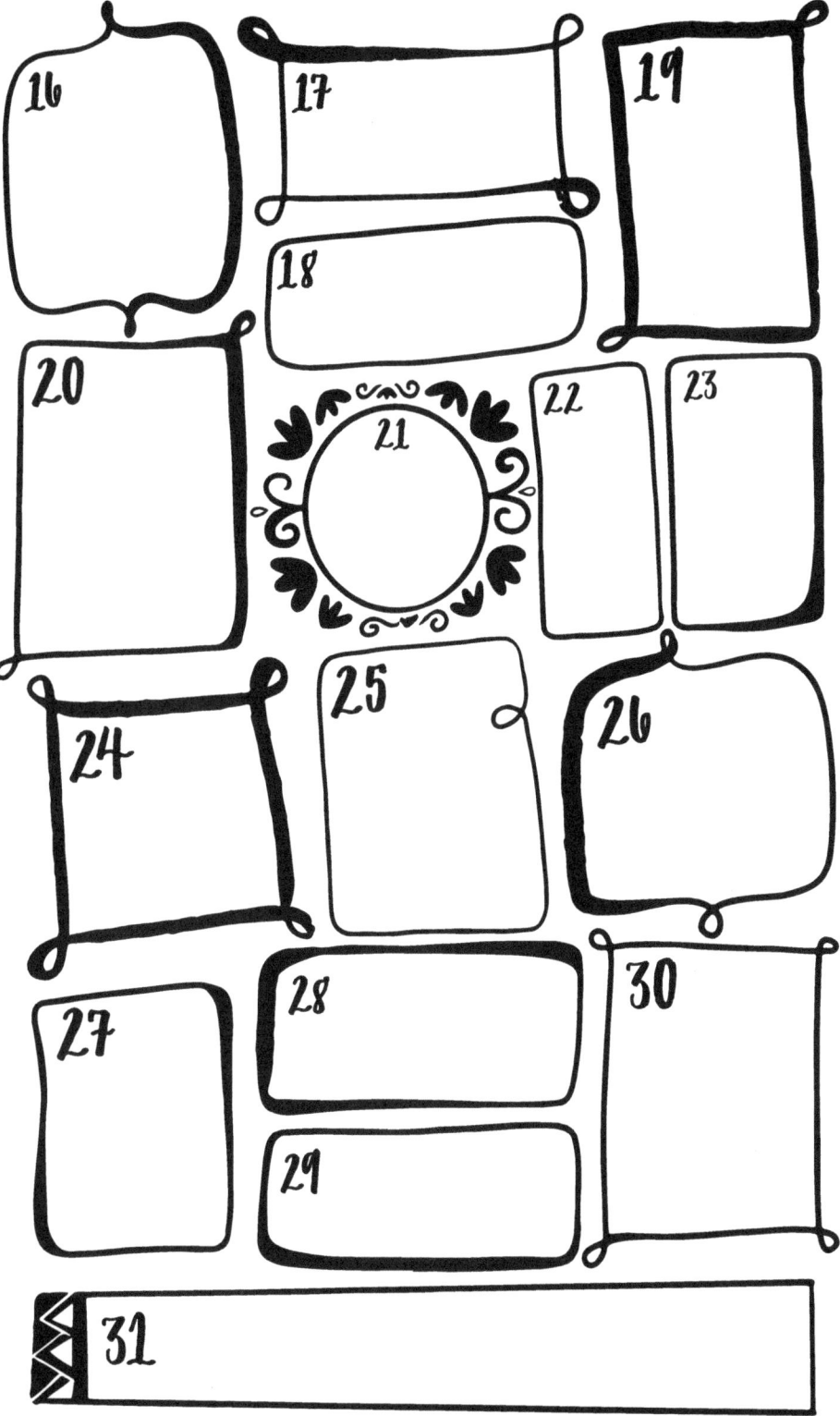

Birthdays, events, notes,

september

1
2
3
4
5
6
7
8
9
10
11
12
13
14
15

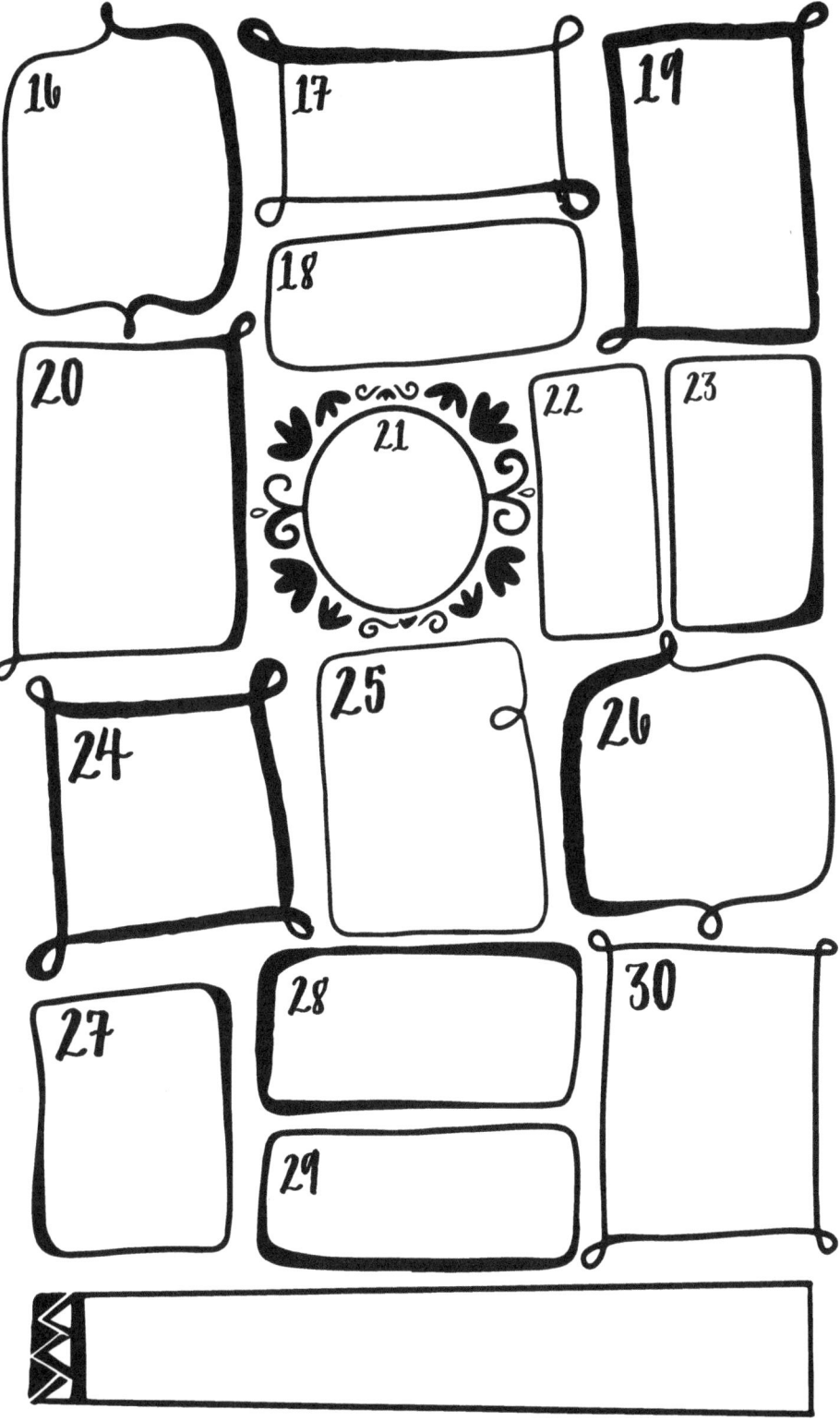

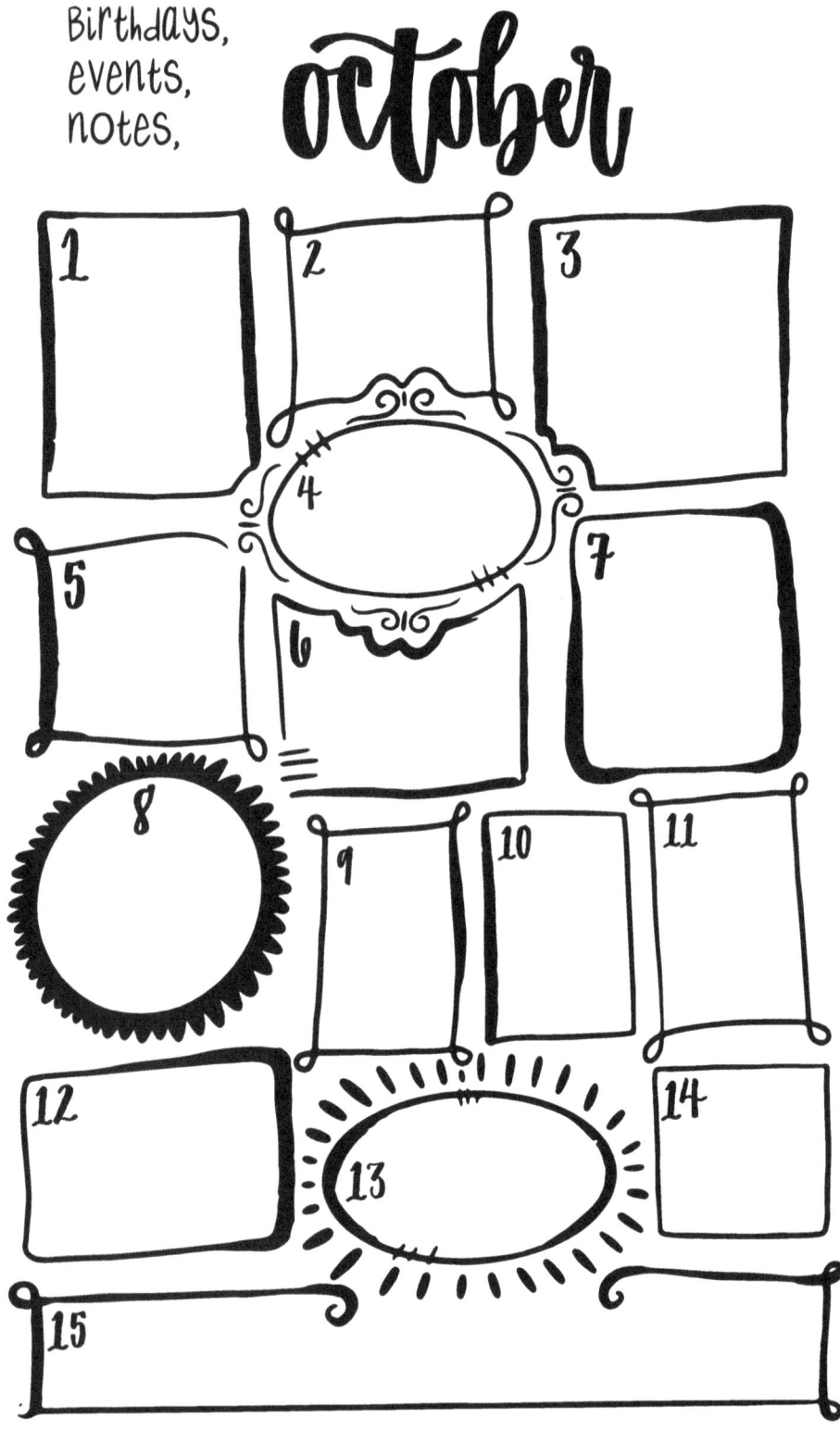

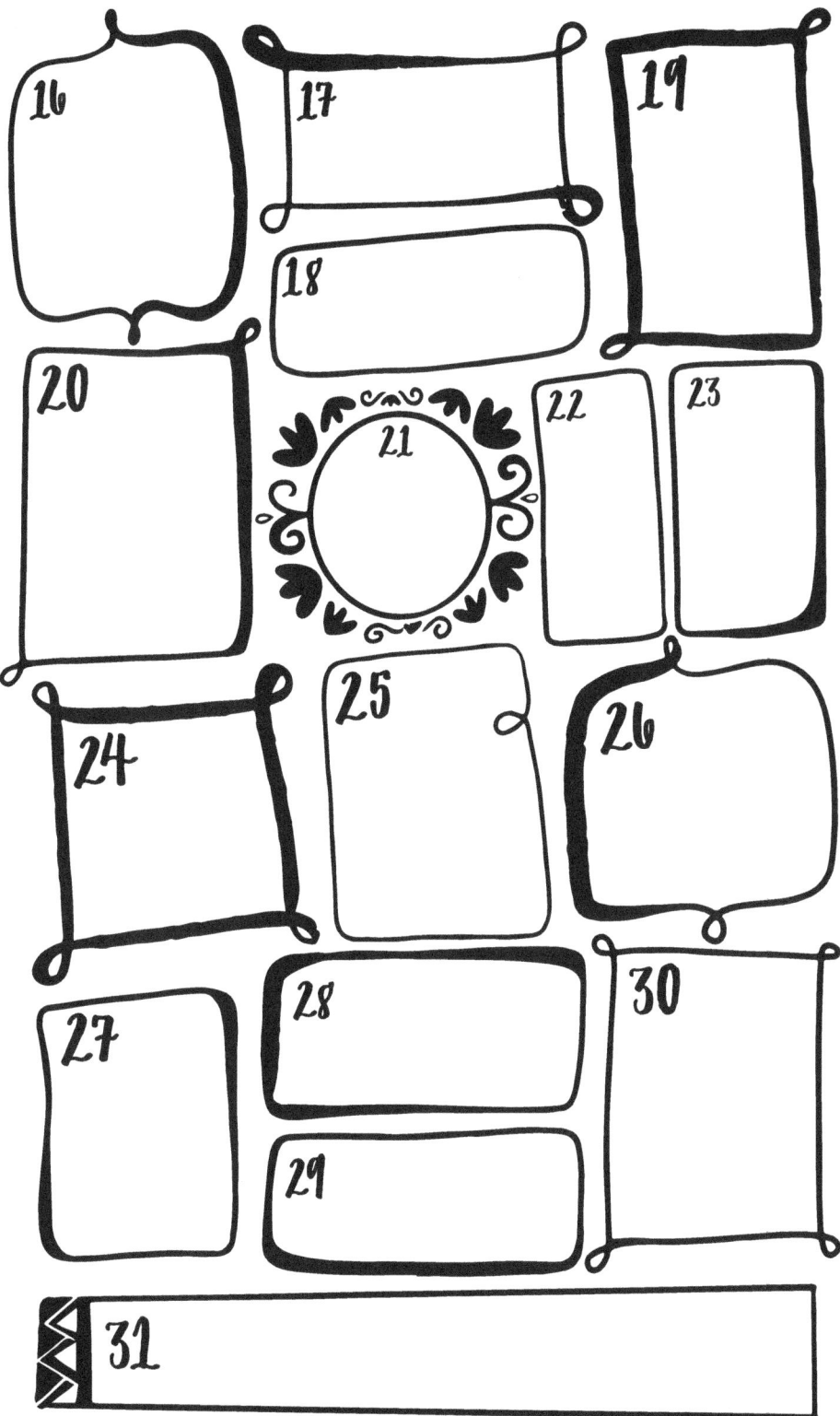

Birthdays, events, notes,

november

1
2
3
4
5
6
7
8
9
10
11
12
13
14
15

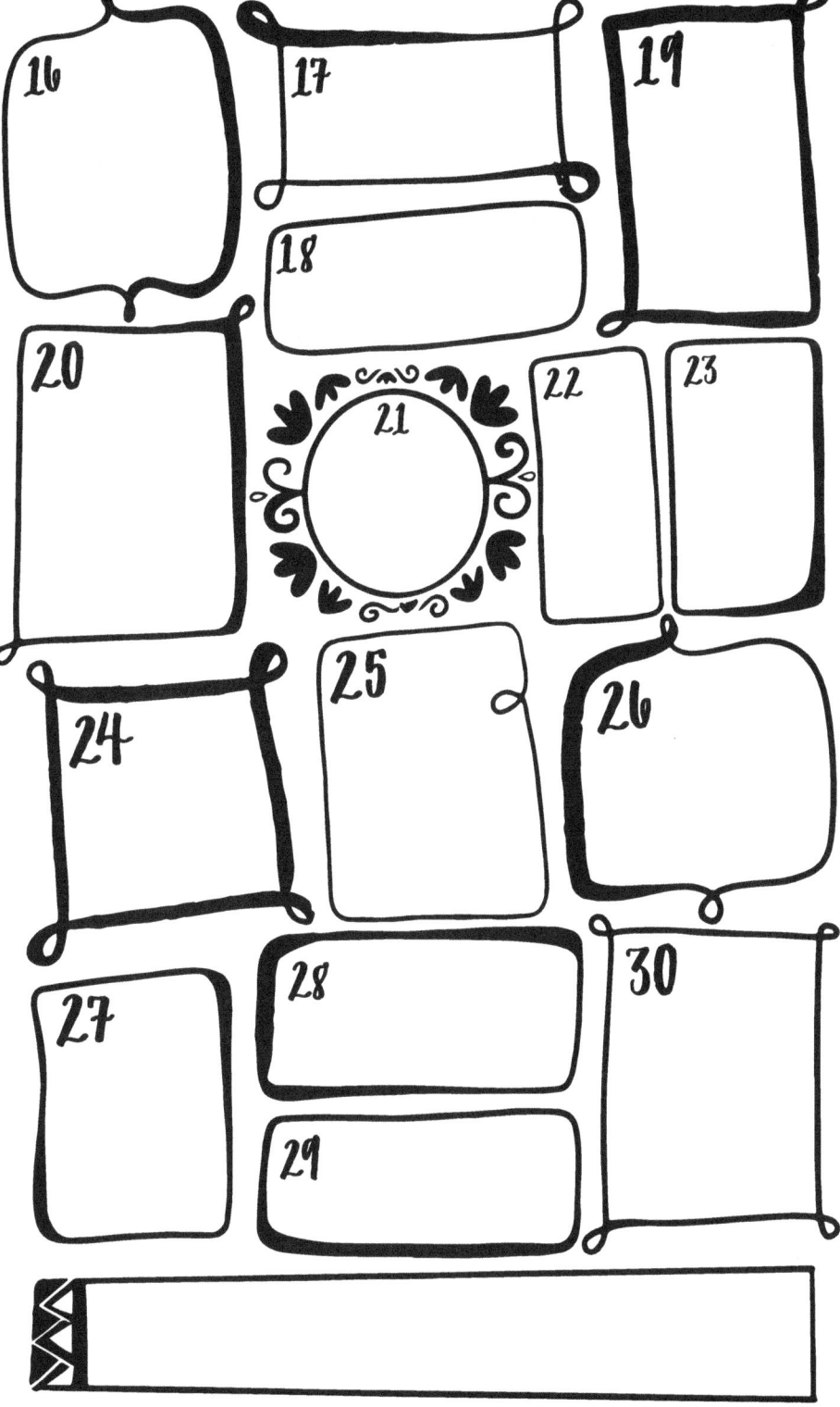

Birthdays, events, notes,

december

1 2 3 4 5 6 7 8 9 10 11 12 13 14 15

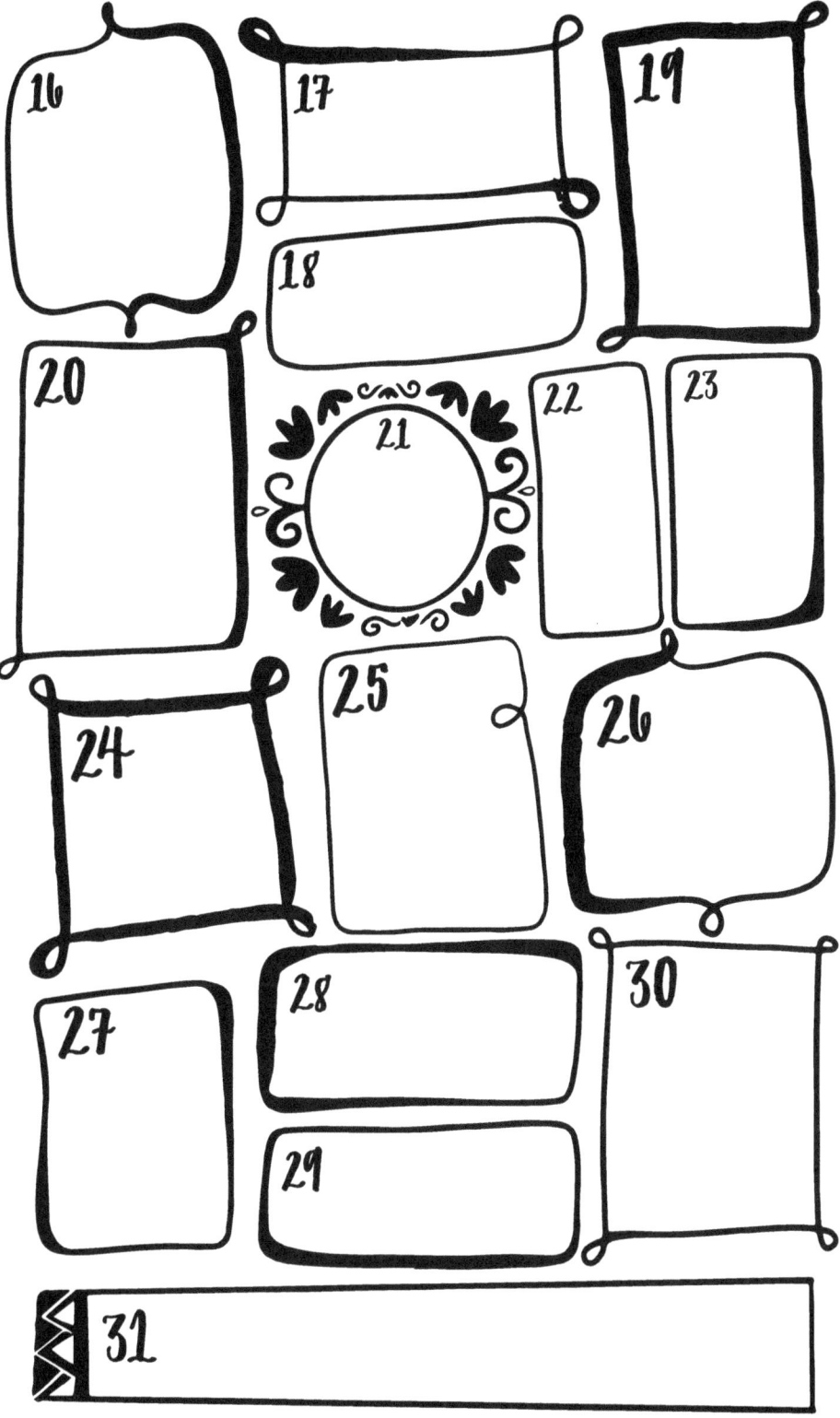

"PEOPLE ARE OFTEN UNREASONABLE, IRRATIONAL, AND SELF-CENTERED. FORGIVE THEM ANYWAY.
IF YOU ARE KIND, PEOPLE MAY ACCUSE YOU OF SELFISH, ULTERIOR MOTIVES. BE KIND ANYWAY.
IF YOU ARE SUCCESSFUL, YOU WILL WIN SOME UNFAITHFUL FRIENDS AND SOME GENUINE ENEMIES. SUCCEED ANYWAY. IF YOU ARE HONEST AND SINCERE PEOPLE MAY DECEIVE YOU. BE HONEST AND SINCERE ANYWAY. WHAT YOU SPEND YEARS CREATING, OTHERS COULD DESTROY OVERNIGHT. CREATE ANYWAY.
IF YOU FIND SERENITY AND HAPPINESS, SOME MAY BE JEALOUS. BE HAPPY ANYWAY. THE GOOD YOU DO TODAY, WILL OFTEN BE FORGOTTEN. DO GOOD ANYWAY. GIVE THE BEST YOU HAVE, AND IT WILL NEVER BE ENOUGH. GIVE YOUR BEST ANYWAY. IN THE FINAL ANALYSIS, IT IS BETWEEN YOU AND GOD.
IT WAS NEVER BETWEEN YOU AND THEM ANYWAY.

~MOTHER TERESA"

"And perhaps what made her beautiful was not her appearance or what she achieved, but in her audacity to believe no matter the darkness around her light ran wild within her, and that was the way she came alive, and it showed up in everything."

MORGAN HARPER NICHOLS

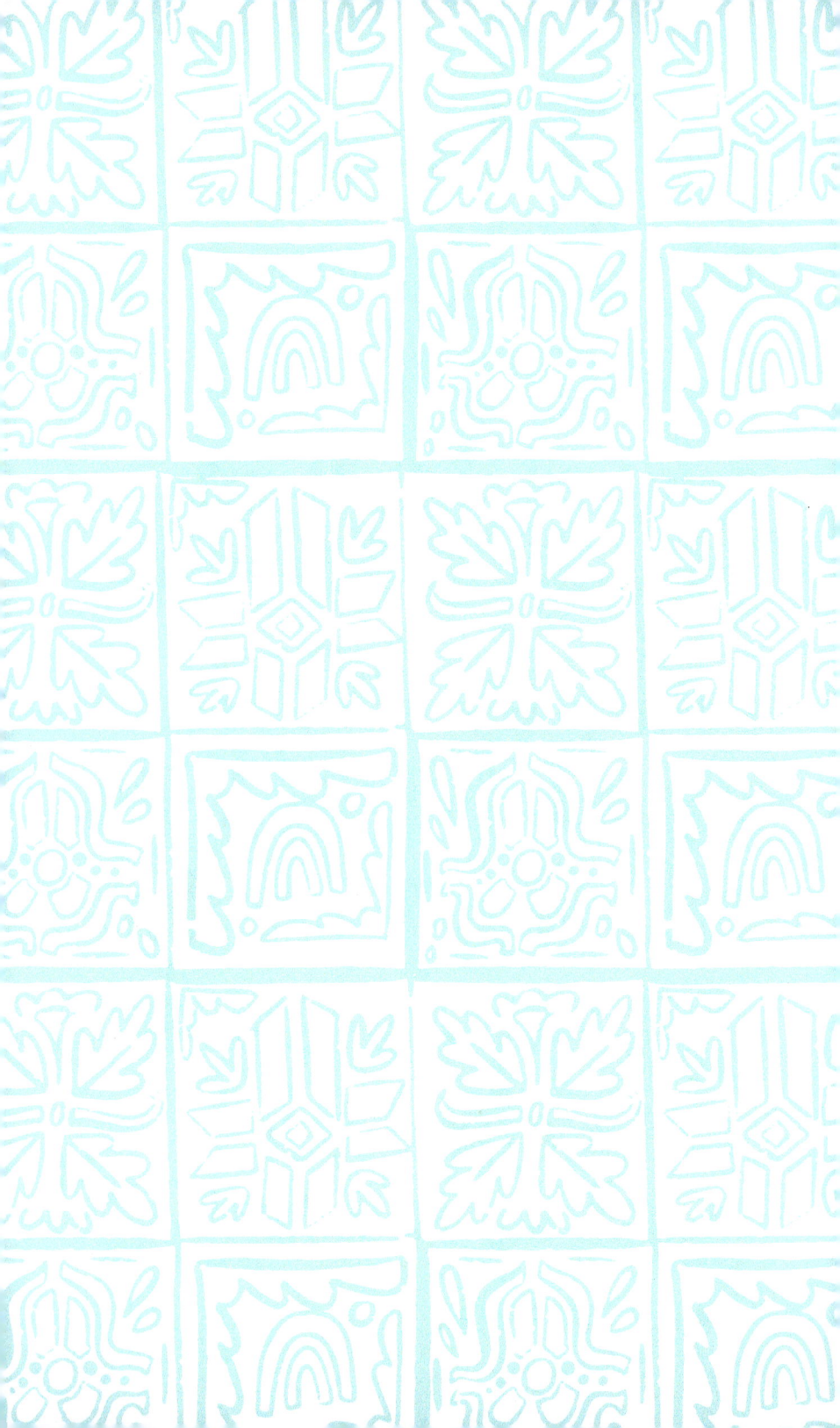

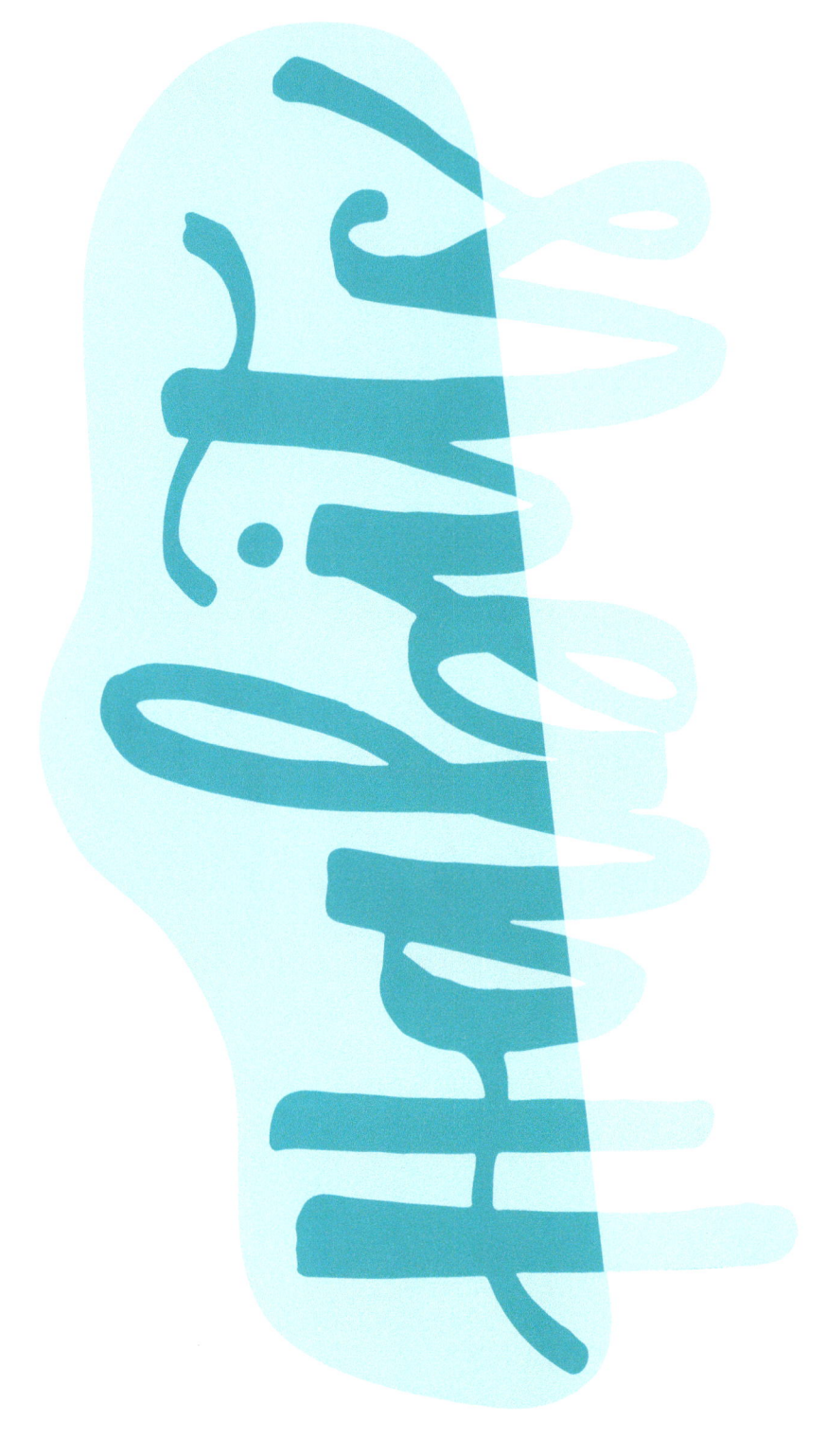

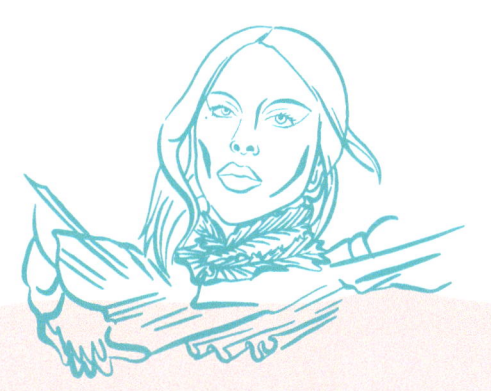

"It's not about how many times you get rejected or fall down or are beaten up, it's about how many times you stand up & are brave & keep on going."

—Lady Gaga

JOY LIST

LIST ALL THINGS THAT MAKE YOU HAPPY.
WHEN YOU'RE SAD, REFLECT ON THE JOY IN YOUR LIFE!

Time Management Skills

Top Ten Tips

1. Pre plan your days by creating a to do list
2. Prioritize what's important
3. Group similar tasks
4. Complete the biggest tasks first
5. Minimize distracting things
6. Be accountable
7. Delegate tasks!
8. Create "me time" for yourself
9. Keep your eye on the prize
10. Manage stress by taking short meditation breaks!

Read more here:

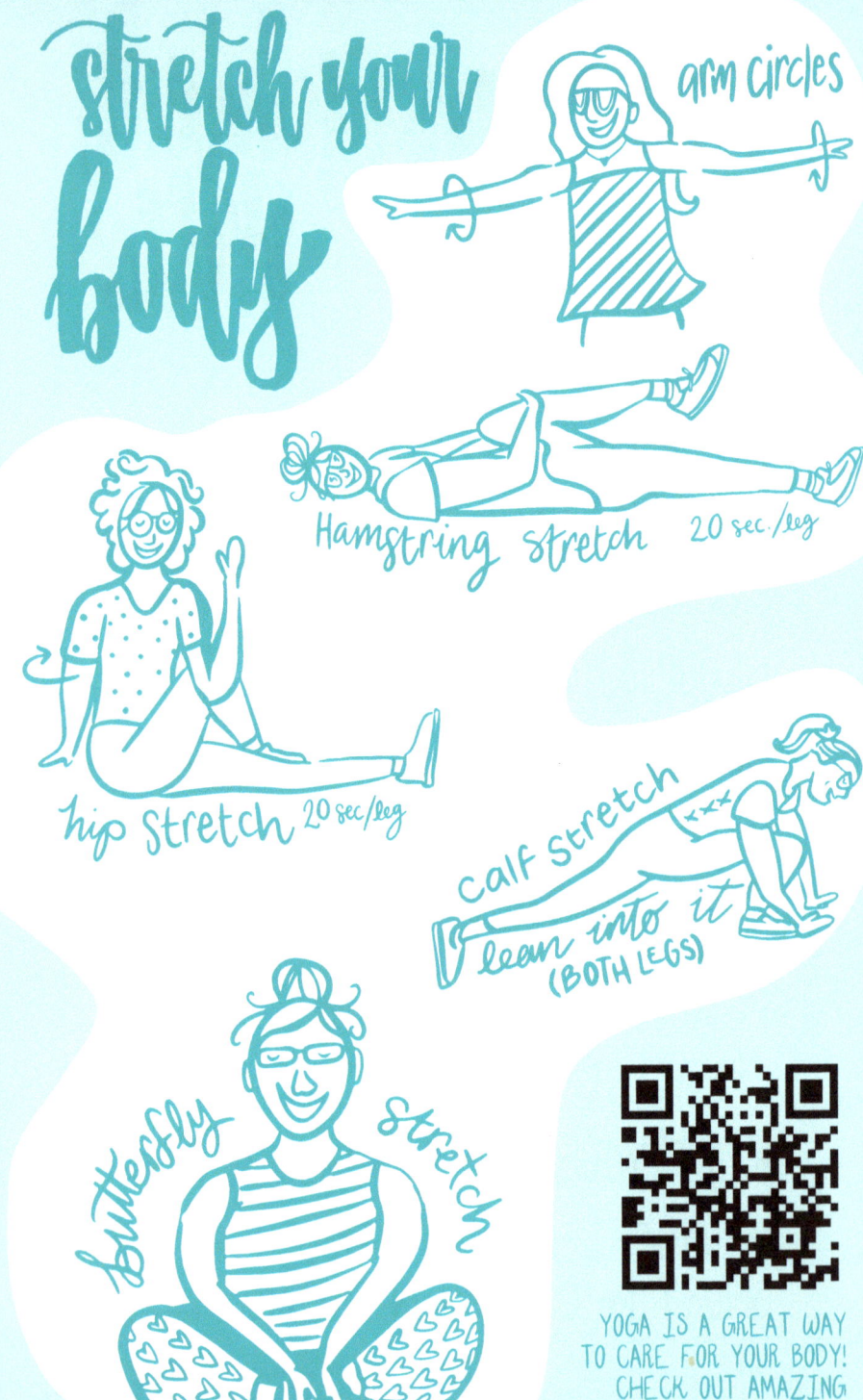

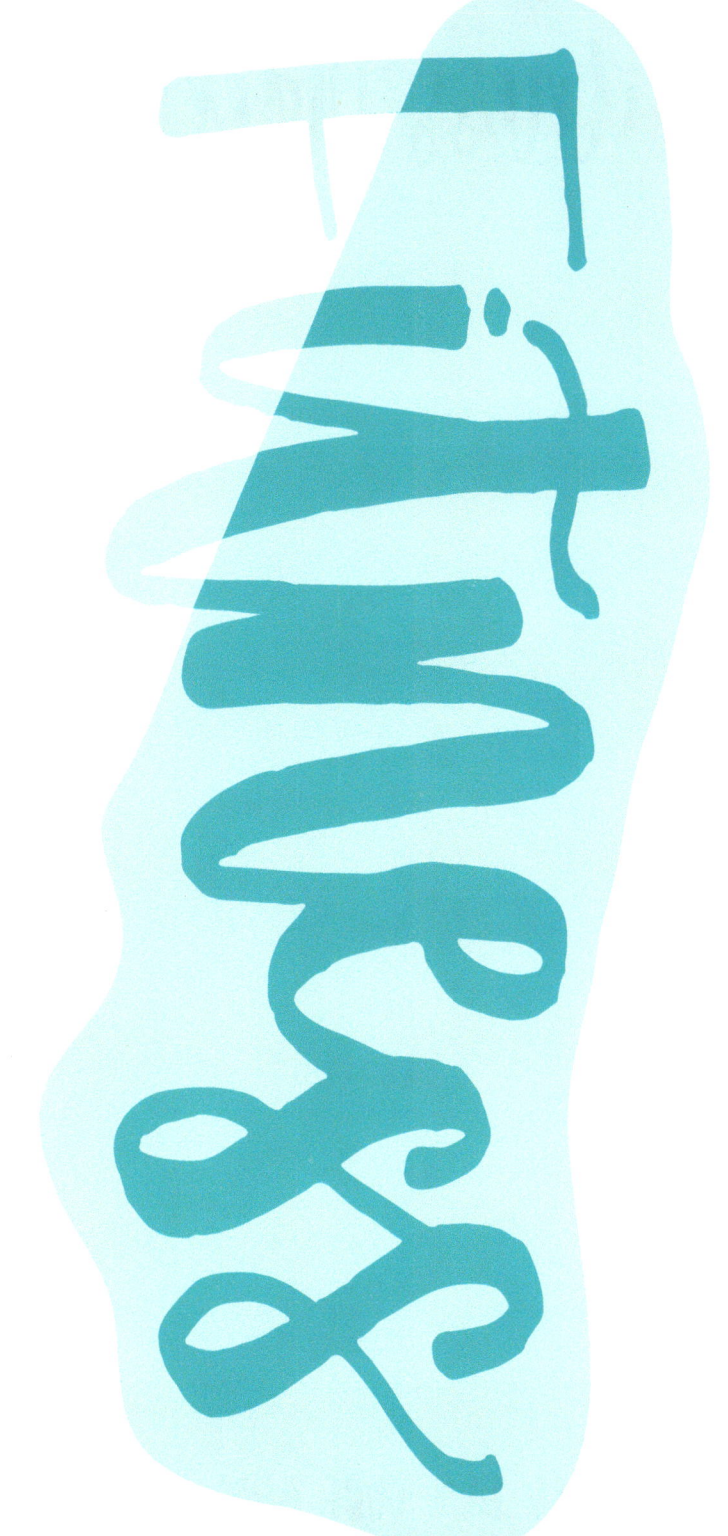

Fitness tracker

color code:
CARDIO WALK RUN CORE ARMS BIKE YOGA

Fitness tracker

color code:
CARDIO WALK RUN CORE ARMS BIKE YOGA

Fitness Tracker

color code:
CARDIO WALK RUN CORE ARMS BIKE YOGA

Fitness Tracker

color code:
CARDIO WALK RUN CORE ARMS BIKE YOGA

Fitness tracker

color code: CARDIO WALK RUN CORE ARMS BIKE YOGA

Fitness tracker

color code:
CARDIO WALK RUN CORE ARMS BIKE YOGA

Fitness tracker

color code:
CARDIO WALK RUN CORE ARMS BIKE YOGA

Fitness tracker

color code: CARDIO WALK RUN CORE ARMS BIKE YOGA

Fitness tracker

minutes: 10 20 30 40 50 60

days: 1-31

color code: CARDIO WALK RUN CORE ARMS BIKE YOGA

Fitness tracker

color code:
CARDIO WALK RUN CORE ARMS BIKE YOGA

Draw/map it Out

Workout: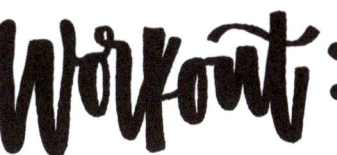

duration:

reminders
- DID YOU STRETCH?
- DID YOU DRINK ENOUGH WATER
- WHAT PLAYLIST DID YOU LISTEN TO?
  _____
  _____

notes:

Draw/map it out

Workout:

_____

_____

duration:

_____

reminders
- DID YOU STRETCH?
- DID YOU DRINK ENOUGH WATER
- WHAT PLAYLIST DID YOU LISTEN TO?

_____

_____

notes:

draw/map it out

Workout:

_____

_____

duration:

reminders
- DID YOU STRETCH?
- DID YOU DRINK ENOUGH WATER
- WHAT PLAYLIST DID YOU LISTEN TO?

_____

_____

notes:

draw/map it out

workout: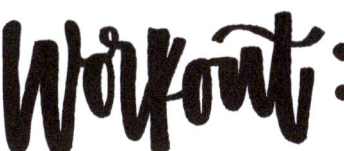

duration:

reminders
- DID YOU STRETCH?
- DID YOU DRINK ENOUGH WATER
- WHAT PLAYLIST DID YOU LISTEN TO?
  _____
  _____

notes:

Draw/map it Out

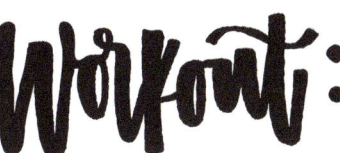

Workout:

duration:

reminders
- DID YOU STRETCH?
- DID YOU DRINK ENOUGH WATER
- WHAT PLAYLIST DID YOU LISTEN TO?
  _____
  _____

notes:

draw/map it out

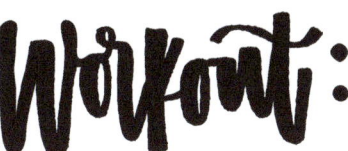

duration:

reminders
- DID YOU STRETCH?
- DID YOU DRINK ENOUGH WATER
- WHAT PLAYLIST DID YOU LISTEN TO?
- _____
- _____

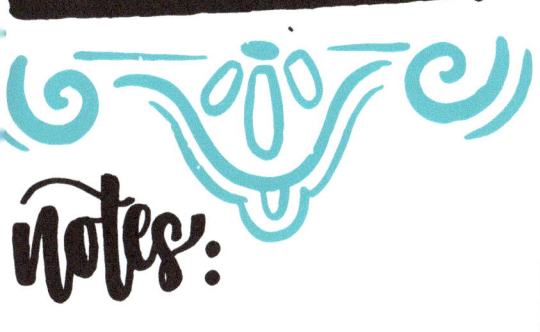

notes:

Draw/map it out

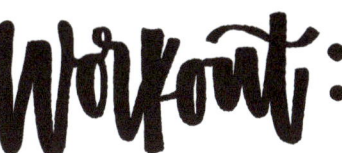
Workout:

duration:

notes:
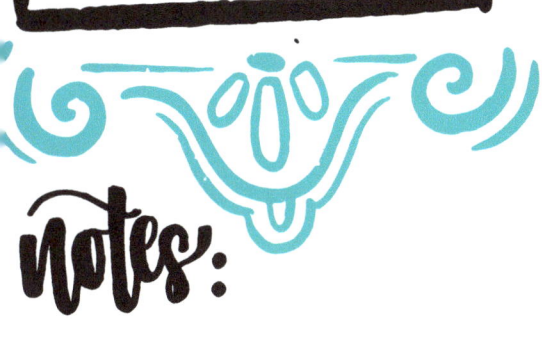

reminders
- DID YOU STRETCH?
- DID YOU DRINK ENOUGH WATER
- WHAT PLAYLIST DID YOU LISTEN TO?

_____
_____

Draw/map it out

Workout:

_____
_____
_____

duration:

_____
_____

reminders
- DID YOU STRETCH?
- DID YOU DRINK ENOUGH WATER
- WHAT PLAYLIST DID YOU LISTEN TO?

_____
_____

notes:

Draw/map it Out

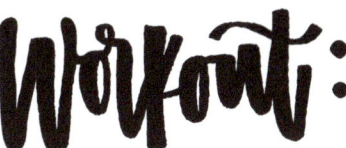

duration:

reminders
- DID YOU STRETCH?
- DID YOU DRINK ENOUGH WATER
- WHAT PLAYLIST DID YOU LISTEN TO?

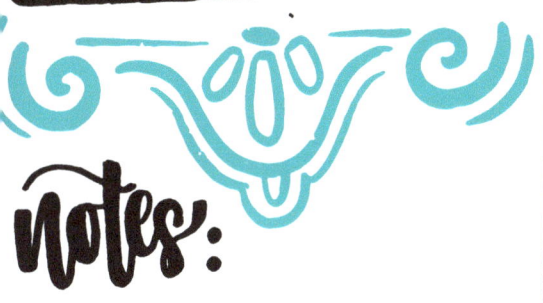

notes:

Draw/map it out

Workout:

duration:

reminders
- DID YOU STRETCH?
- DID YOU DRINK ENOUGH WATER
- WHAT PLAYLIST DID YOU LISTEN TO?
  _____
  _____

notes:

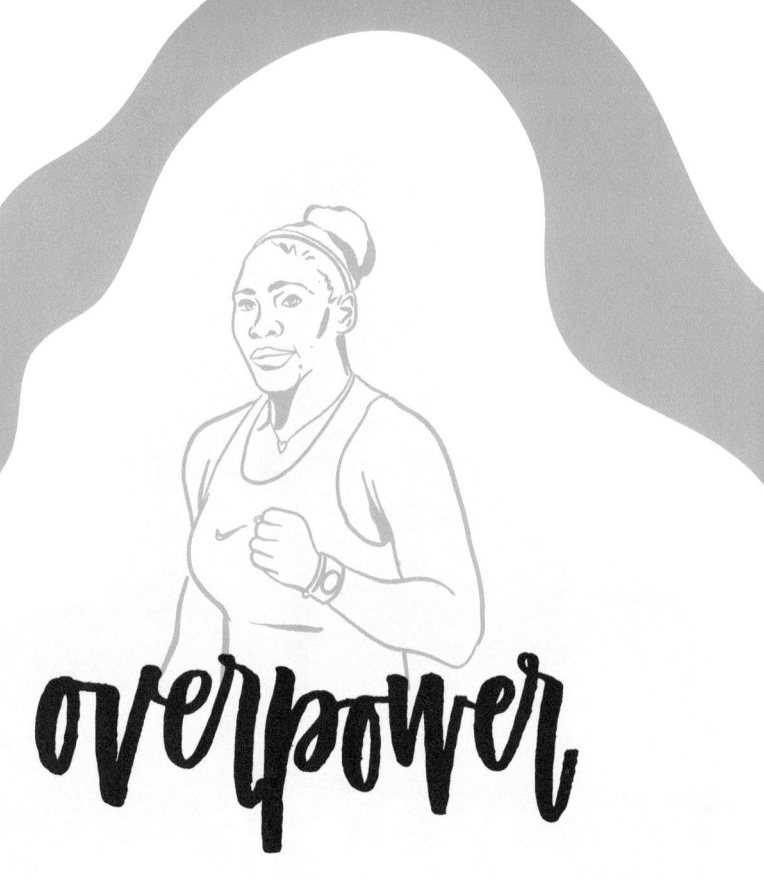

overpower

SERENA WILLIAMS

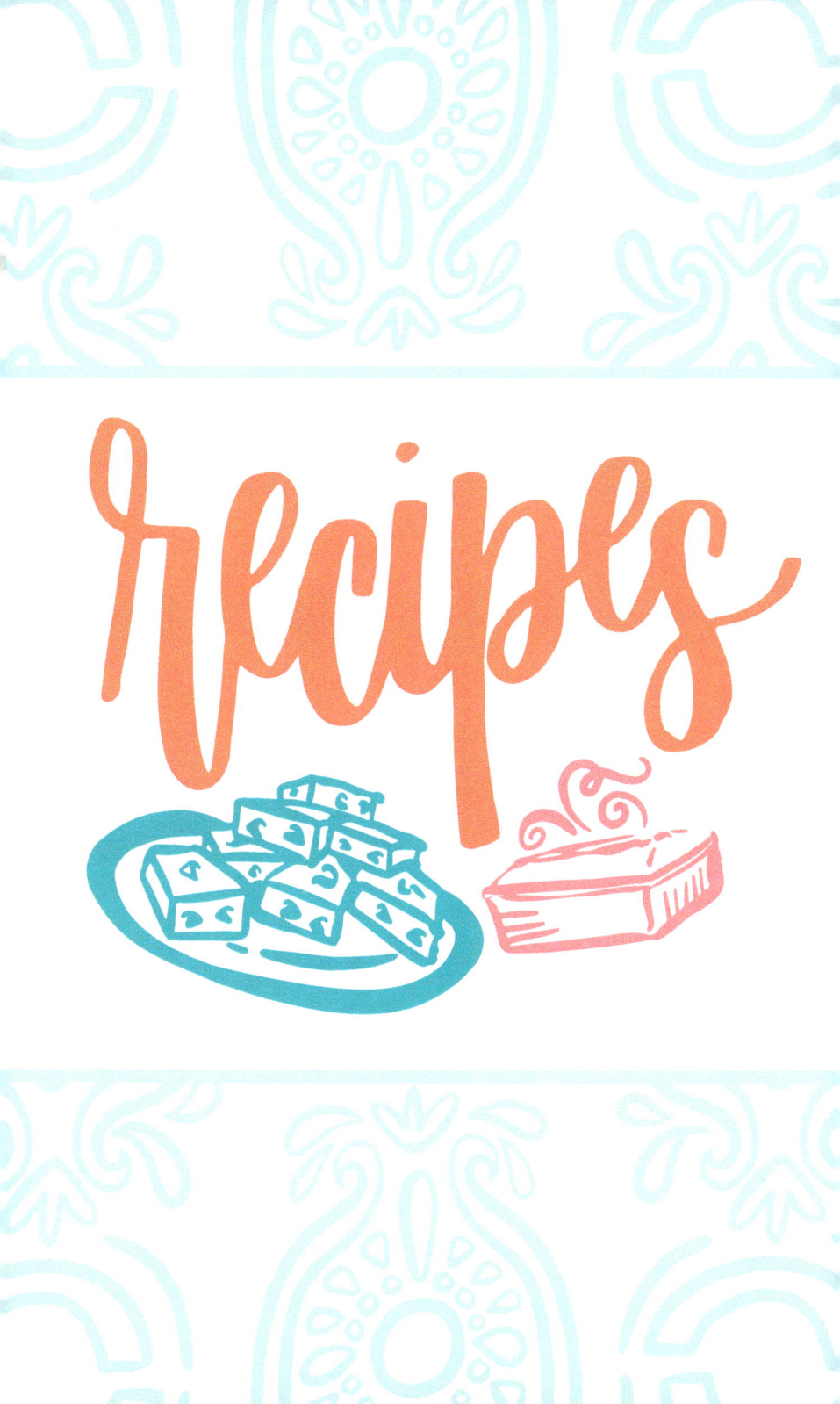

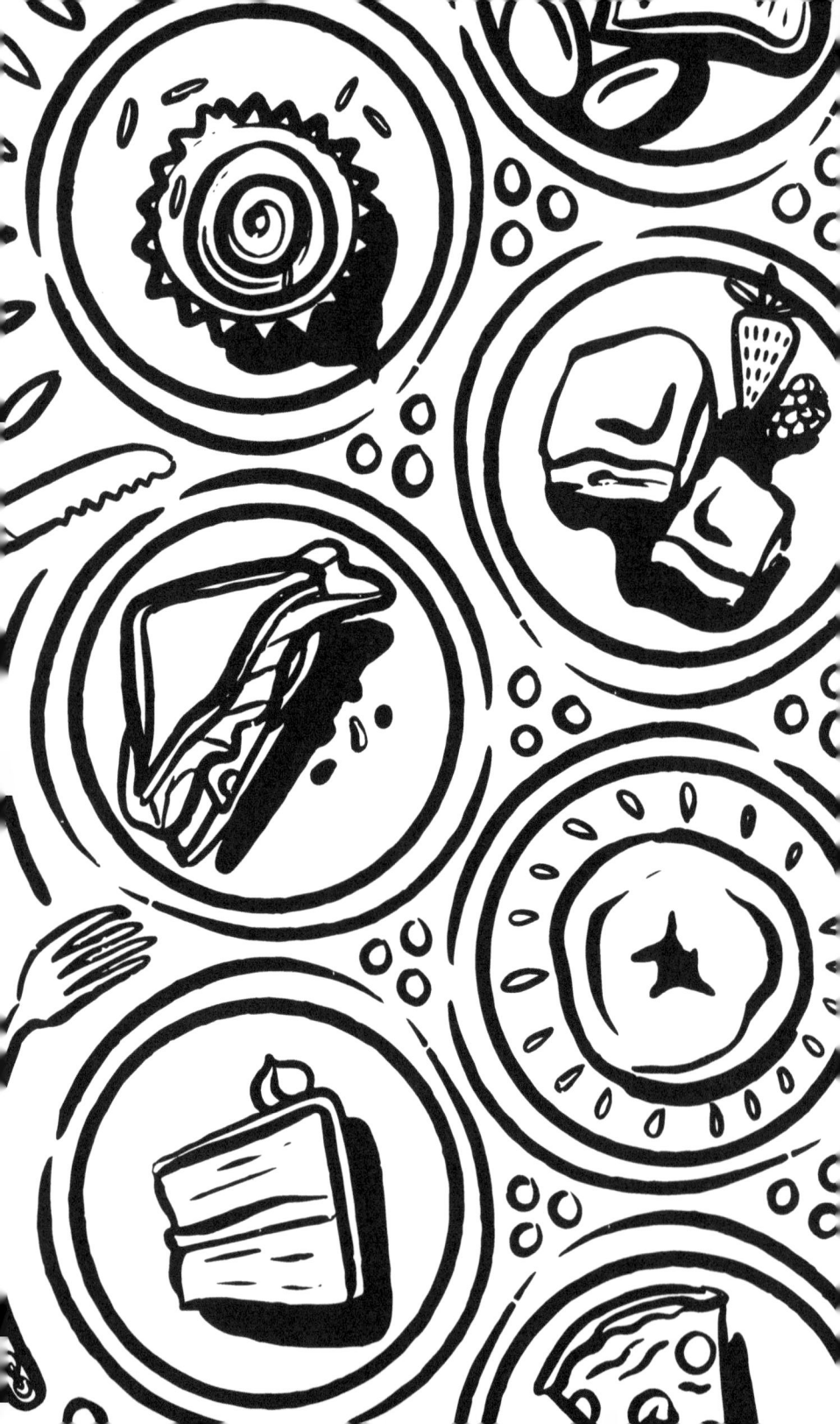

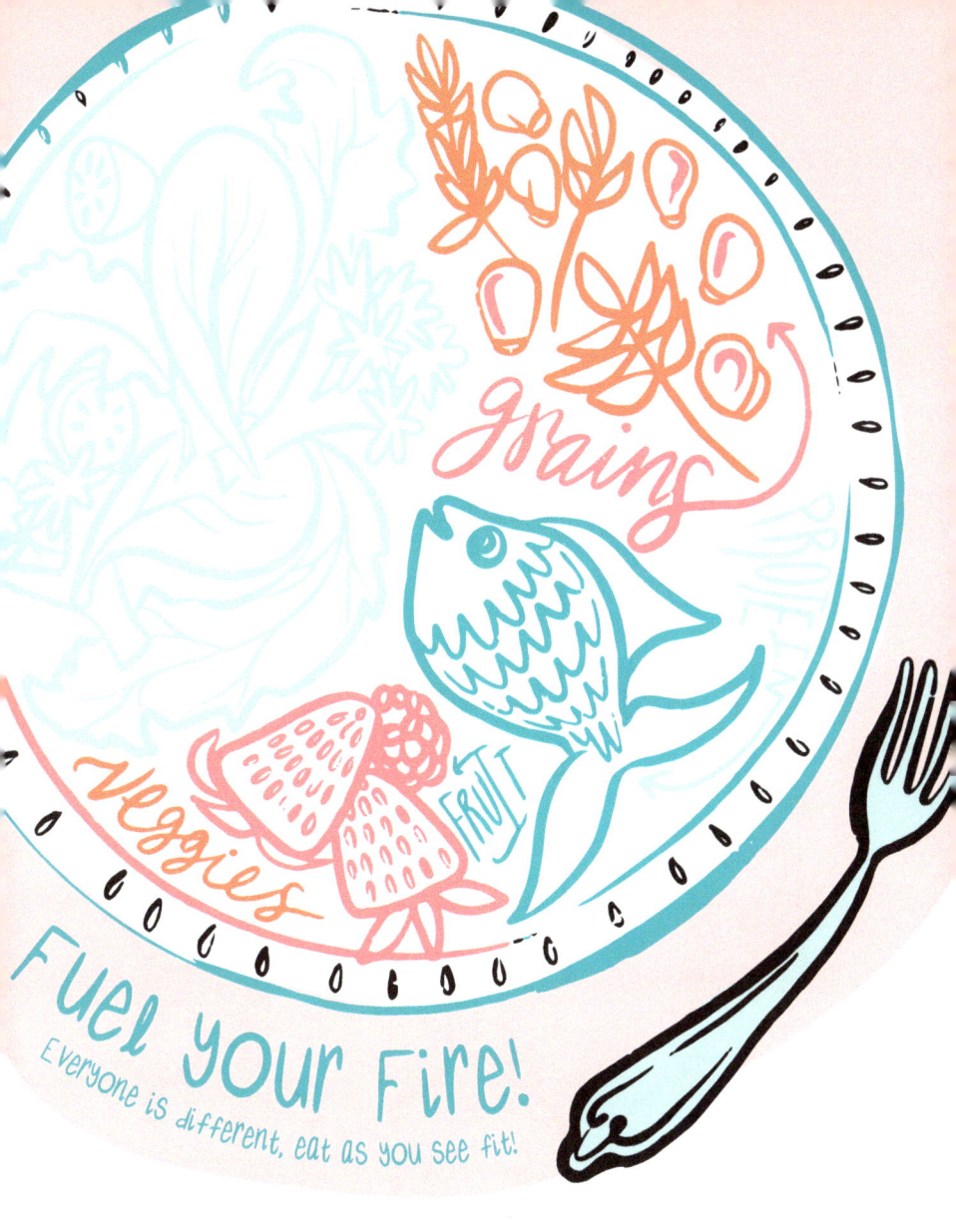

TRY TO INCORPORATE COLOR THROUGH FRUITS AND VEGGIES!
FIND YOUR BALANCE BETWEEN CARBS, PROTEINS, AND HEALTHY FATS!

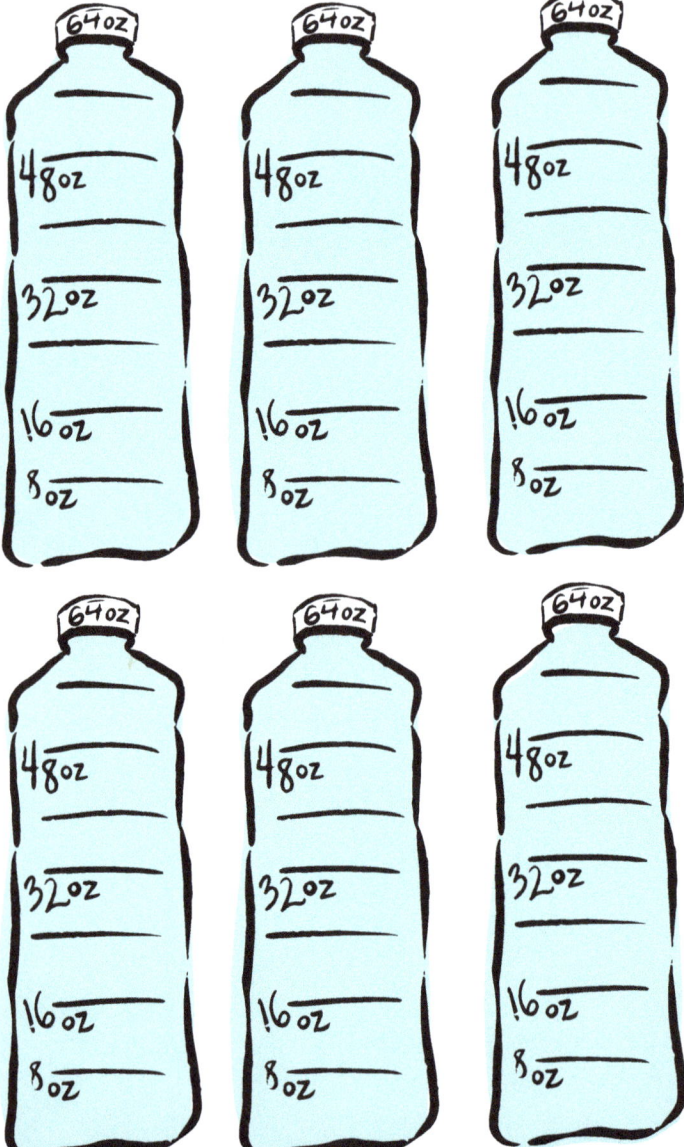

COMMON CONVERSIONS

Measurement:	cup	Tablespoon	ounces	grams
Butter	1 cup	16 Tbsp	8 oz	227g
Sifted Flour	1 cup	16 Tbsp	4.24/3.88 oz	120-110g
Granulated Sugar	1 cup	16 Tbsp	7 oz	200g
Packed Brown Sugar	1 cup	16 Tbsp	6.4 oz	180g
Water	1 cup	16 Tbsp	8 oz	227g

NEED TO KNOW CONVERSIONS:

1 TBSP = 3 tsp
4 TBSP = ¼ cup
1 cup = 250 mL
1 pint = 500 mL
1 quart = 0.95 L
1 gallon = 3.8 L

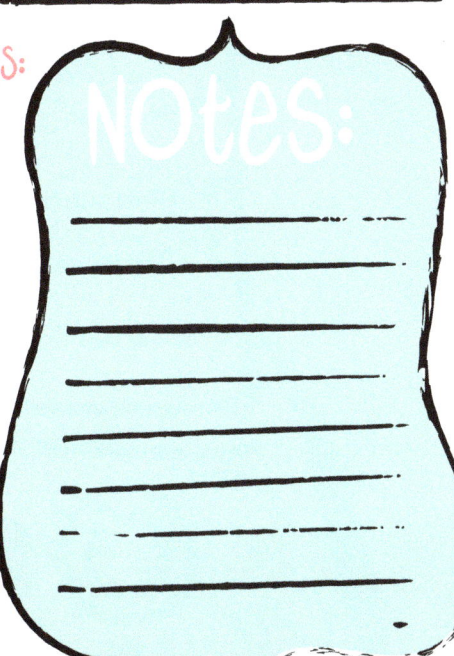

NOTES:

THE BERRY BEST SMOOTHIE GUIDE

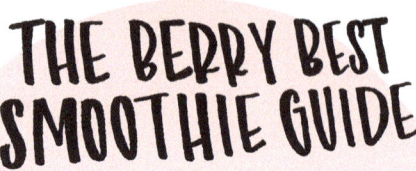

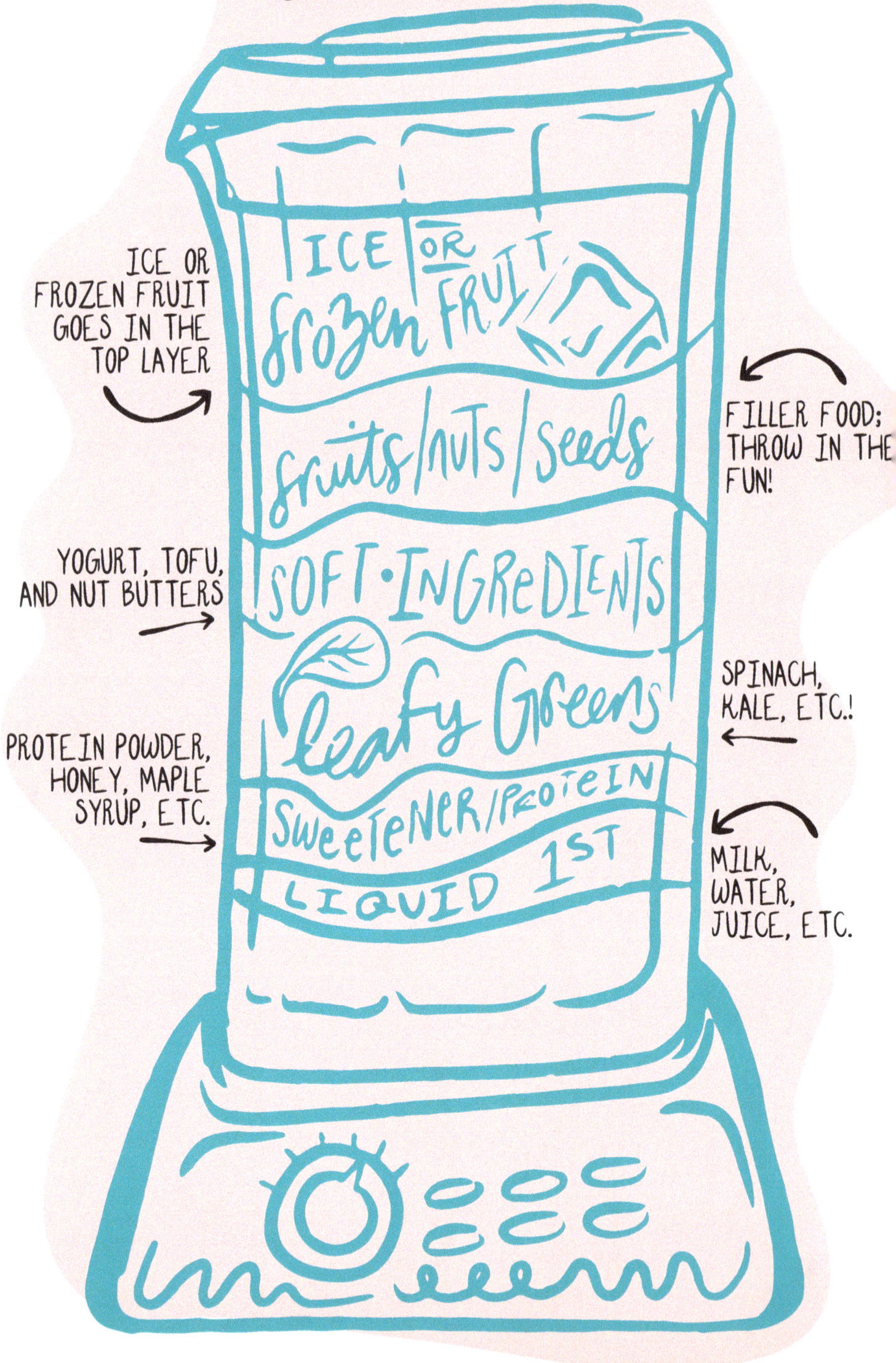

SMOOTHIE IDEAS

1. CHOOSE A BASE: A CUP OF LIQUID
2. TROW IN SOME GREENS: TWO CUPS
3. ADD FROZEN FRUIT: ONE TO TWO CUPS
4. BOOST WITH PROTEIN: ONE HALF CUP OF YOGURT, PROTEIN POWDER
5. THROW IN SOME HEALTHY FATS: ONE TO TWO TBS OF NUT BUTTERS OR HANDFUL OF NUTS
6. SWEETEN IF YOU'E FEELING SPUNKY: ONE TSP OF MAPLE SYRUP OR HONEY
7. EXTRA ADD-INS: ONE TO TWO TBS OF COCOA POWDER, NUTRIONAL POWDERS, SEEDS AND NUTS, NUT BUTTERS

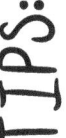

TIPS:

IF YOU DON'T HAVE FROZEN FRUIT, USE FRESH AND THROW IN SOME ICE CUBES TO THICKEN. A COMBO OF FROZEN AND FRESH FRUITS WILL WORK AS WELL!

MORE FROZEN INGEDEINTS : THICKER SMOOTHIE
MORE LIQUID : THINNER SMOOTHIE

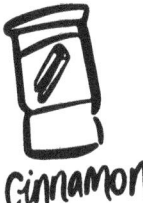
Cinnamon

RECIPE IDEAS:

Strawberry Banana Protein:
- 1 CUP OF UNSWEETENED ALMOND MILK
- 1 1/2 CUPS FROZEN STRAWBERRIES
- 1/2 CUP FROZEN BANANA
- 1/4 CUPS OF VANILLA PROTEIN POWDER
- 1/3 CUP OF NONFAT GREEK YOUGURT

Mixed Berry:
- 1 CUP OF UNSWEETENED MILK
- 2 CUPS OF SPINACH
- 1 CUP OF FROZEN BANANA (SLICED)
- 1 CUP OF FROZEN MIXED BERRIES
- Add Protein Powder or Sweetener if desired

Peanut Butter Banana:
- 2 CUPS SLICED FROZEN BANANA
- 1 CUPS OF SPINACH
- 2 TBS OF PROTEIN POWDER
- 2 CUPS OF ALMOND MILK

Peach Pie Smoothie:
- 1/2 CUP OF FROZEN BANANA (SLICED)
- 1 PEACH
- 1/2 CUP ALMOND OR RICE MILK
- 1/2 SCOOP OF PROTEIN POWDER (HEMP PREFERRED)
- 1/4 PINCH OF NUTMEG
- 1/4 TSP CINNAMON
- 1/2 CUP ALMONDS
- 1/2 CUP VANILLA YOGURT

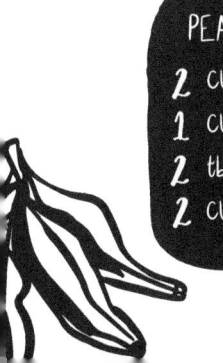

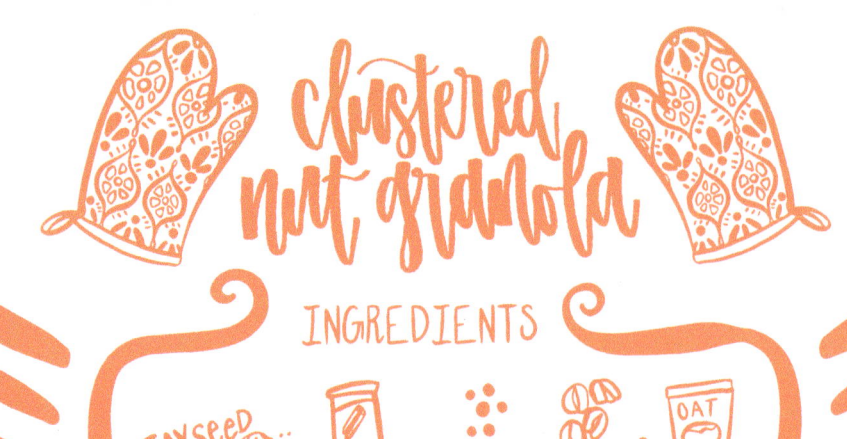

Clustered Nut Granola

INGREDIENTS

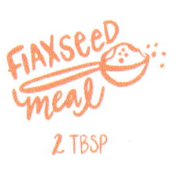 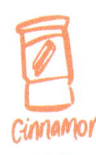 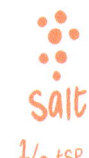 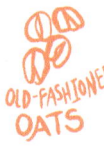 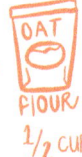

- Flaxseed Meal — 2 TBSP
- Cinnamon — 2 tsp
- Salt — 1/2 tsp
- Old-Fashioned Oats — 2 cups
- Oat Flour — 1/2 cup

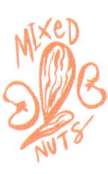 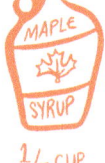 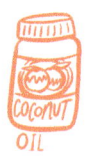 

- Mixed Nuts — 2 cups
- Maple Syrup — 1/3 cup
- Coconut Oil — 1/4 cup
- Vanilla — 1 tsp

INSTRUCTIONS

1. Preheat the oven to 300° degrees and line a large baking sheet with parchment paper.
2. Combine dry ingredients. In a separate bowl whisk together wet ingredients. Add wet ingredients to dry ingredients. Ensure it's thoroughly mixed and oats are completely coated.
3. Spread on parchment paper covered baking sheet and bake for 20-35 minutes. May need to stir outer sections of the oats to avoid burning.
4. Granola is finished baking when it appears slightly golden brown. Be careful it will burn easily.
5. Let cool before breaking apart. Store in an airtight container and enjoy!

Perfect pairing with milk, yogurt, or enjoy by itself.

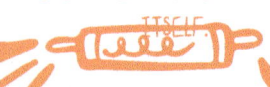

Recipe

TITLE: _____

INGREDIENTS
_____
_____
_____
_____
_____
_____
_____
_____

Picture Of Recipe

INSTRUCTIONS: _____
_____
_____
_____
_____
_____
_____
_____

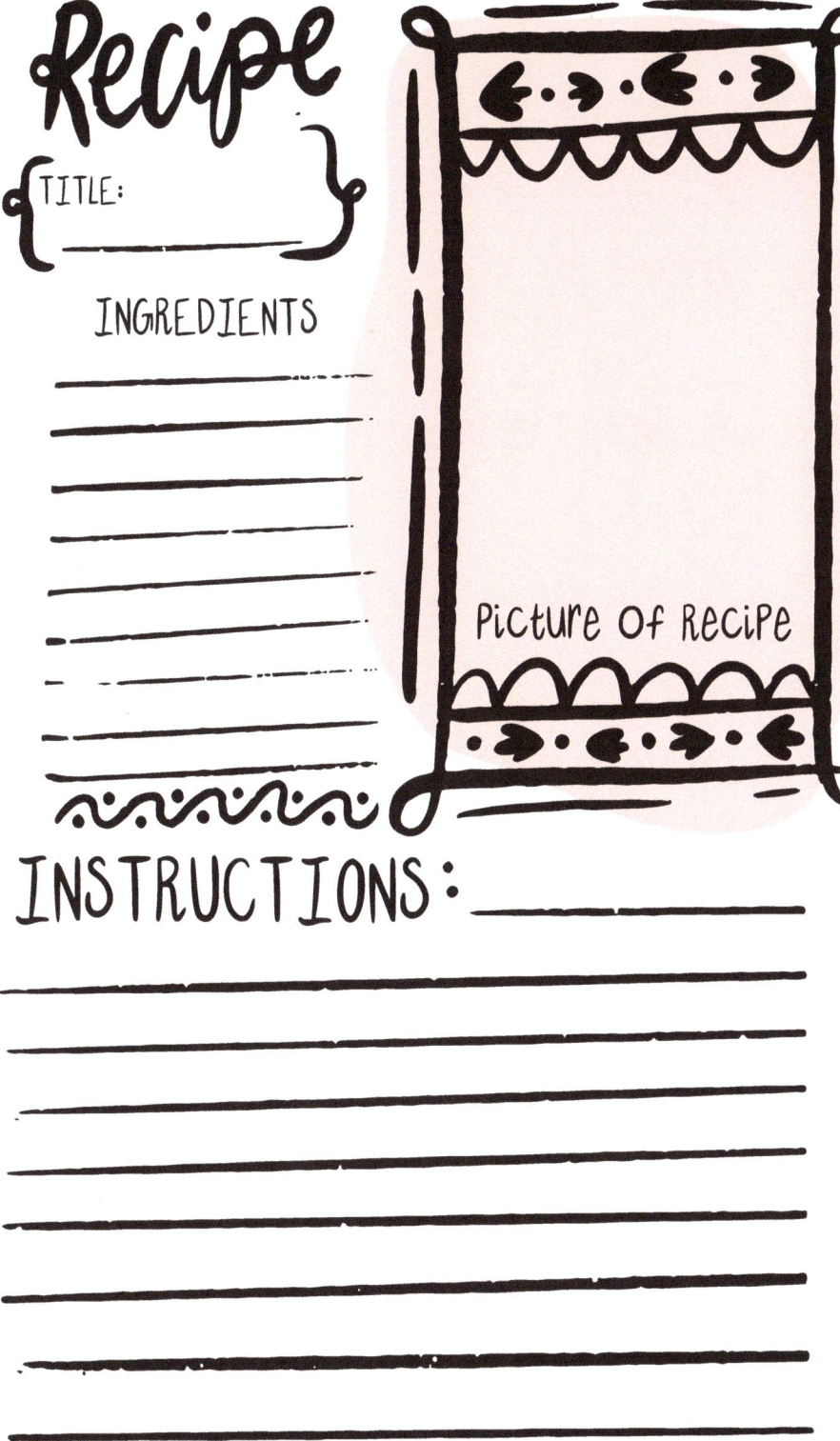

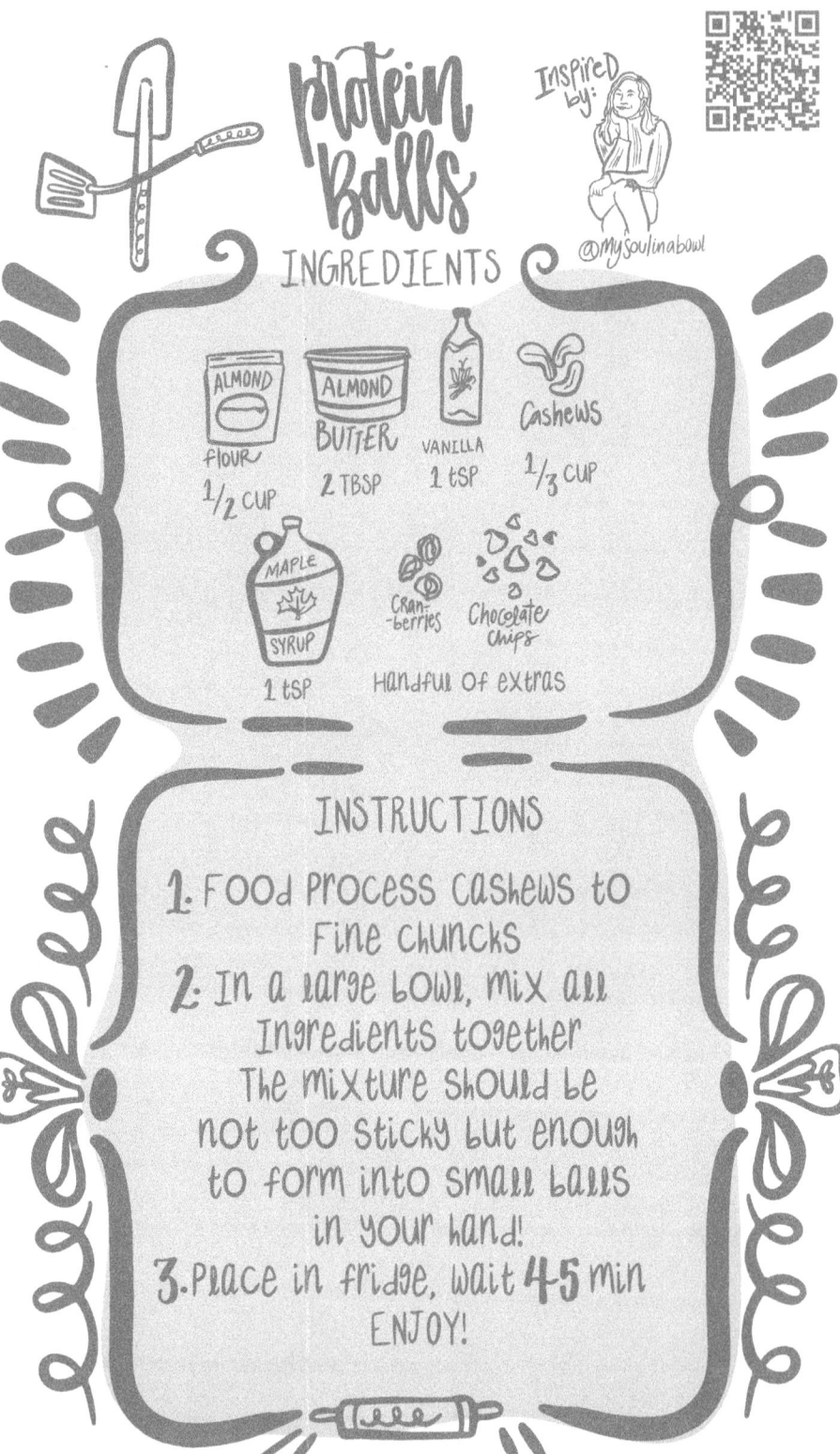

Recipe

{ TITLE: _____ }

INGREDIENTS
_____
_____
_____
_____
_____
_____
_____

Picture Of Recipe

INSTRUCTIONS: _____
_____
_____
_____
_____
_____
_____
_____
_____

Banana Bread

INGREDIENTS

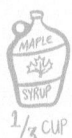
Maple Syrup
1/3 cup

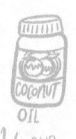
Coconut Oil
1/3 cup

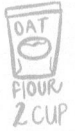
Oat Flour
2 cup

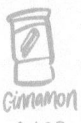
Cinnamon
1 tsp

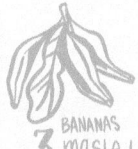
3 Bananas mashed

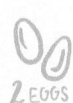
2 Eggs

Baking Powder
1 tsp

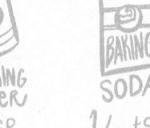
Baking Soda
1/2 tsp

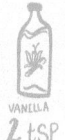
Vanilla
2 tsp

INSTRUCTIONS

1. Preheat the oven to **350°** degrees.
2. Combine bananas and wet ingredients in a bowl.
3. In another bowl mix dry ingredients.
4. Combine wet and dry ingredients, pour into a greased loaf pan and bake for **45** min.
5. Feel free to add nuts, fruit, or other fun ingredients.

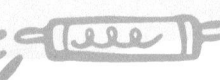

Recipe

{ TITLE: _____ }

INGREDIENTS

_____
_____
_____
_____
_____
_____

Picture Of Recipe

INSTRUCTIONS: _____

_____
_____
_____
_____
_____
_____
_____

sandwich fun

HOW TO BUILD A GOOD SANDWICH:

1. START WITH YOUR BREAD
2. ADD CONDIMENTS
3. THROW IN SOME VEGGIES
4. TOP WITH CHEESE:
5. SPICE IT UP WITH FLAVOR
6. FINISH WITH PROTEIN AND FOLD TOGETHER

Breakfast idea:

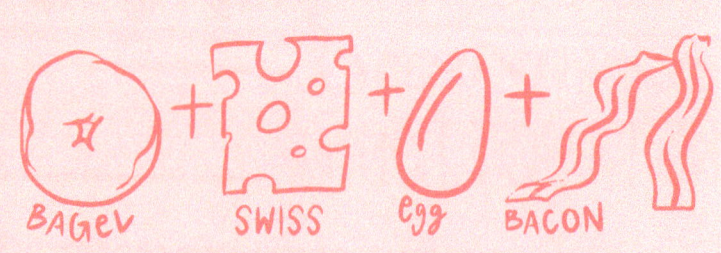

BAGEL + SWISS + EGG + BACON

Lunch idea:

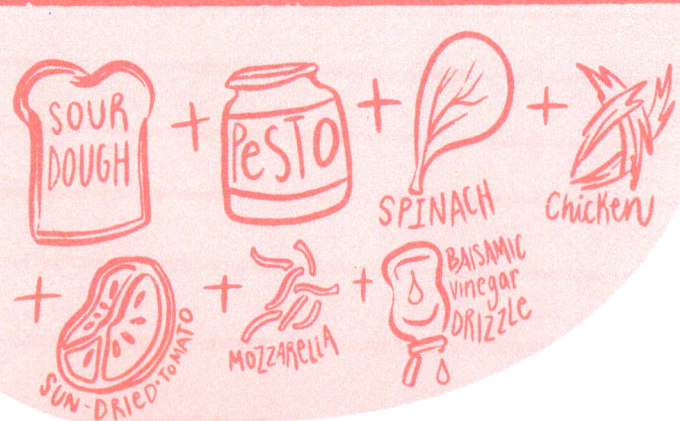

SOUR DOUGH + PESTO + SPINACH + CHICKEN + SUN-DRIED TOMATO + MOZZARELLA + BALSAMIC VINEGAR DRIZZLE

Recipe

TITLE: _____

INGREDIENTS

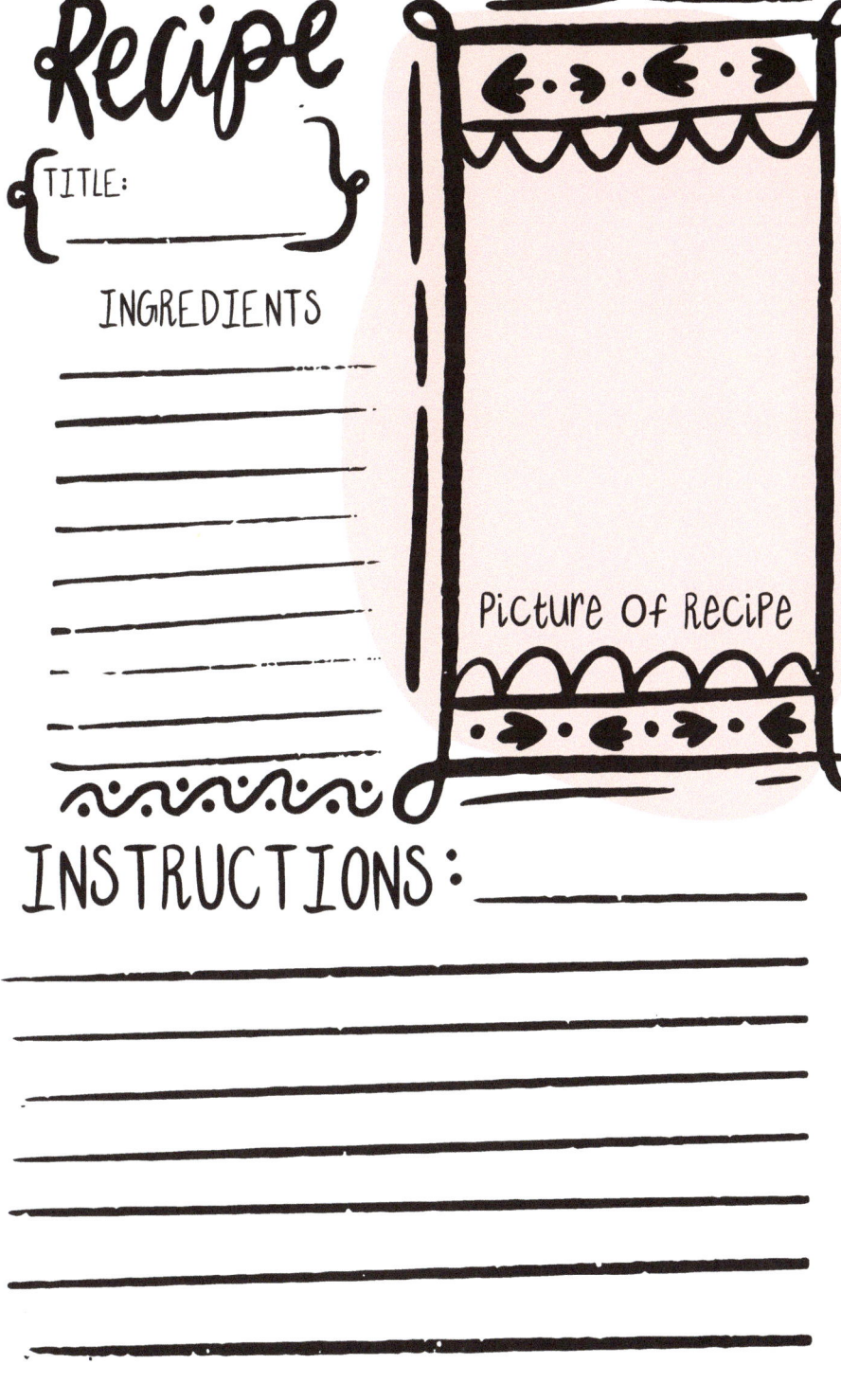

Picture Of Recipe

INSTRUCTIONS: _____

Roasted Veggie Guide:

COAT VEGGIES IN OLIVE OIL, SALT AND PEPPER, AND BAKE AT **425°** FOR THE ALLOTTED TIME AND ENJOY. KEEP IN MIND EVERY OVEN VARIES, SO TIME IS JUST FOR GUIDANCE.

10-15 min.

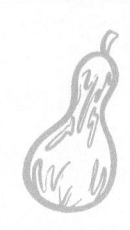
summer squash

15-20 min.

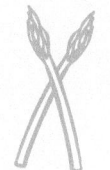 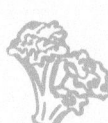
asparagus, broccoli

20-25 min.

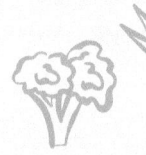 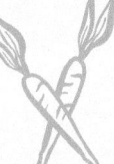 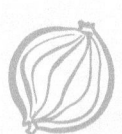 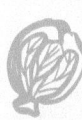
cauliflower, carrots, onions, brussel sprouts

25-30 min.

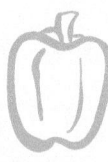 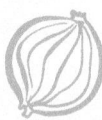
peppers, onions

40-45 min.

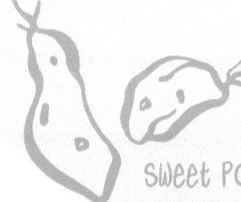
sweet potatoes, white potatoes

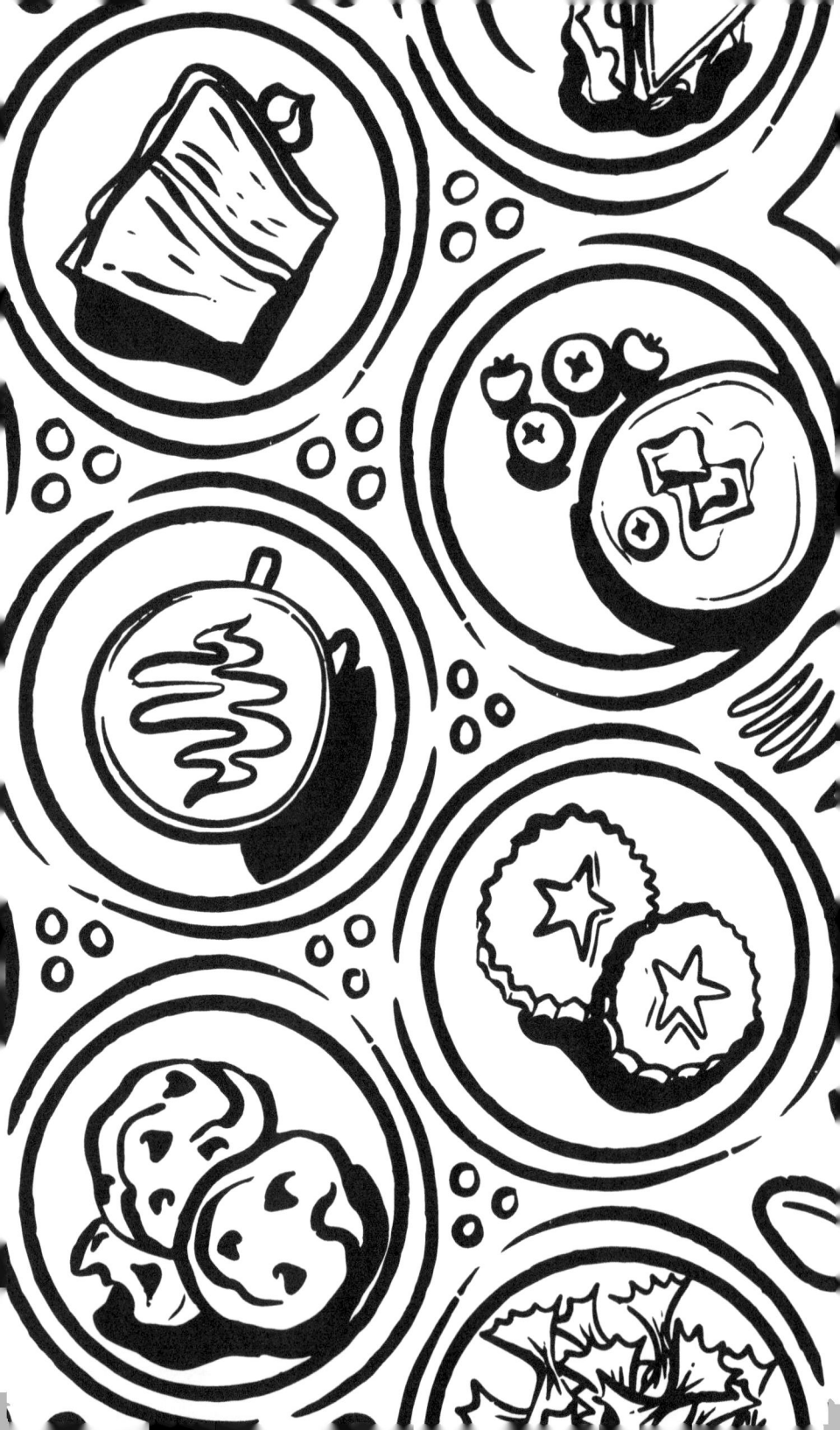

Recipe

TITLE: _____

INGREDIENTS

_____
_____
_____
_____
_____
_____
_____
_____

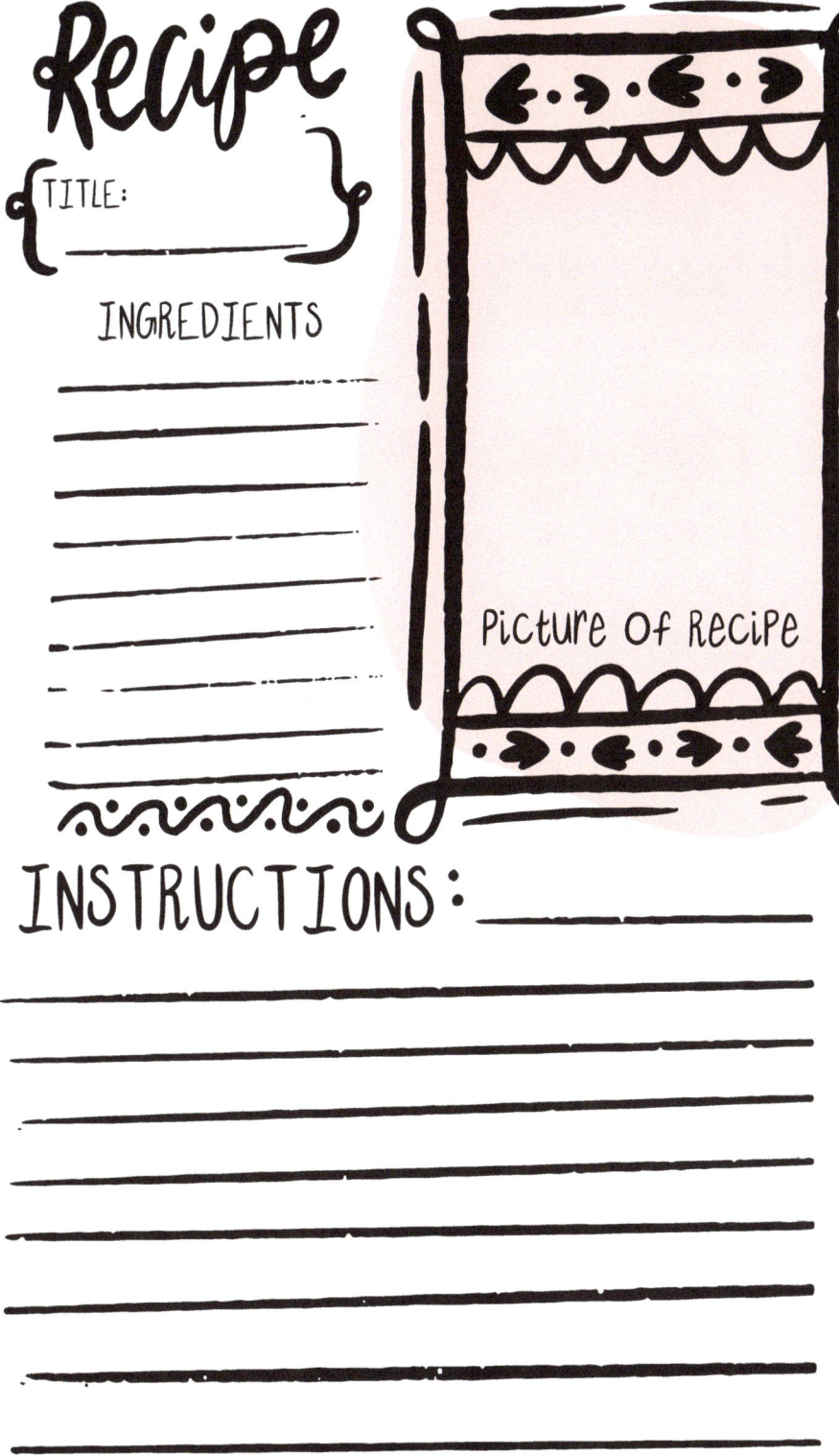

Picture Of Recipe

INSTRUCTIONS: _____

_____
_____
_____
_____
_____
_____
_____
_____
_____

Healthy Brownies

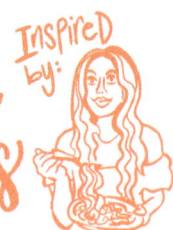 Inspired by:

@hungry.blonde

INGREDIENTS

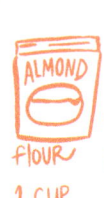 Almond Flour — 1 cup
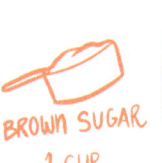 Brown Sugar — 1 cup
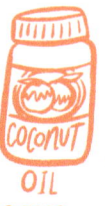 Coconut Oil — 2 tbsp
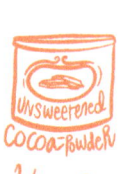 Unsweetened Cocoa Powder — 1/2 cup
 Vanilla — 1 tsp
 Baking Soda — 1/2 tsp
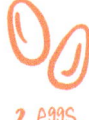 2 eggs
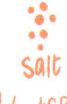 Salt — 1/2 tsp
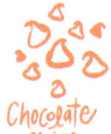 Chocolate Chips

INSTRUCTIONS

1. Mix together all ingredients
2. Fold in chocolate chips
3. Line a 8x8" square baking pan with parchment paper and preheat oven to 350°
4. Bake 25-30 minutes
5. Let cool and ENJOY!!

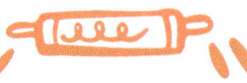

Recipe

TITLE: _____

INGREDIENTS

_____
_____
_____
_____
_____
_____
_____
_____
_____

Picture Of Recipe

INSTRUCTIONS: _____

_____
_____
_____
_____
_____
_____
_____
_____
_____

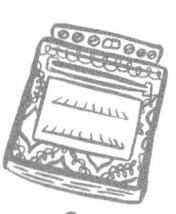
peanut butter blondies

Inspired by:
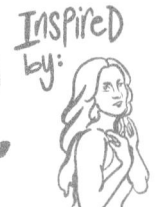
@kalejunkie

INGREDIENTS

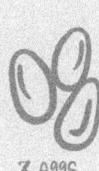 flour 1 3/4 CUP

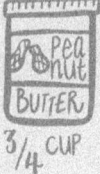 coconut sugar 1 CUP

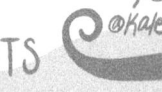 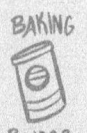  baking powder 2 tsp

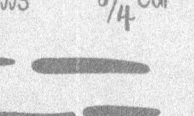 vanilla 1 tsp

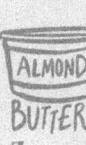 3 eggs

peanut butter 3/4 CUP

almond butter 3/4 CUP

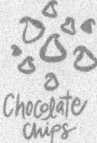 chocolate chips

INSTRUCTIONS

1. Mix together all ingredients
2. Fold in chocolate chips
3. Line a 8x8" square baking pan with parchment paper and preheat oven to 350°
4. Bake just under 25 minutes
5. Let cool and ENJOY!!

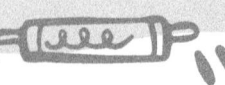

Recipe

TITLE: _____

INGREDIENTS

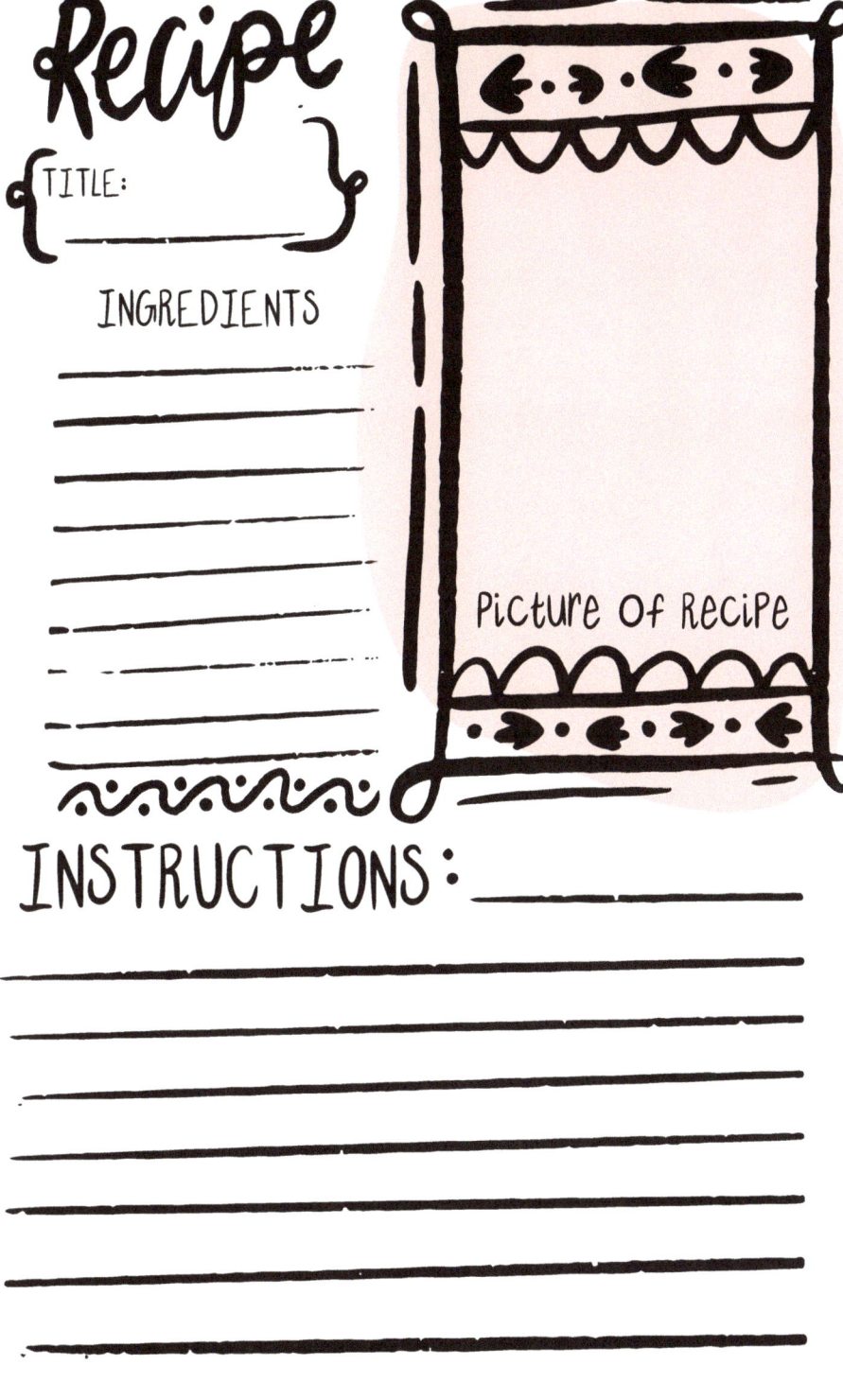

Picture Of Recipe

INSTRUCTIONS: _____

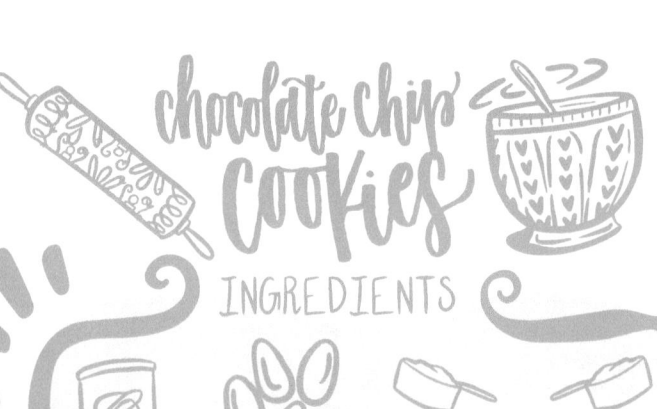

Chocolate Chip Cookies

INGREDIENTS

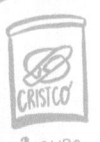   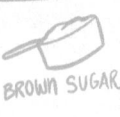

- Cristco — 2 cups
- 4 eggs
- White sugar — 1/2 cup
- Brown sugar — 1/2 cup

   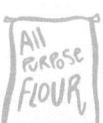 

- Vanilla — 2 tsp
- Baking soda — 2 tsp
- Salt — 2 tsp
- All purpose flour — 4-5 cups
- Chocolate chips — LOTS!

INSTRUCTIONS

1. Preheat the oven to **375°**.
2. Mix all ingredients together ending with the flour and chocolate chips.
3. Place them on a cookie sheet about **1-2"** apart then bake for **10-12** minutes.
4. Let them cool, or eat them warm, and enjoy!

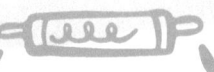

Recipe

{ TITLE: _____ }

INGREDIENTS

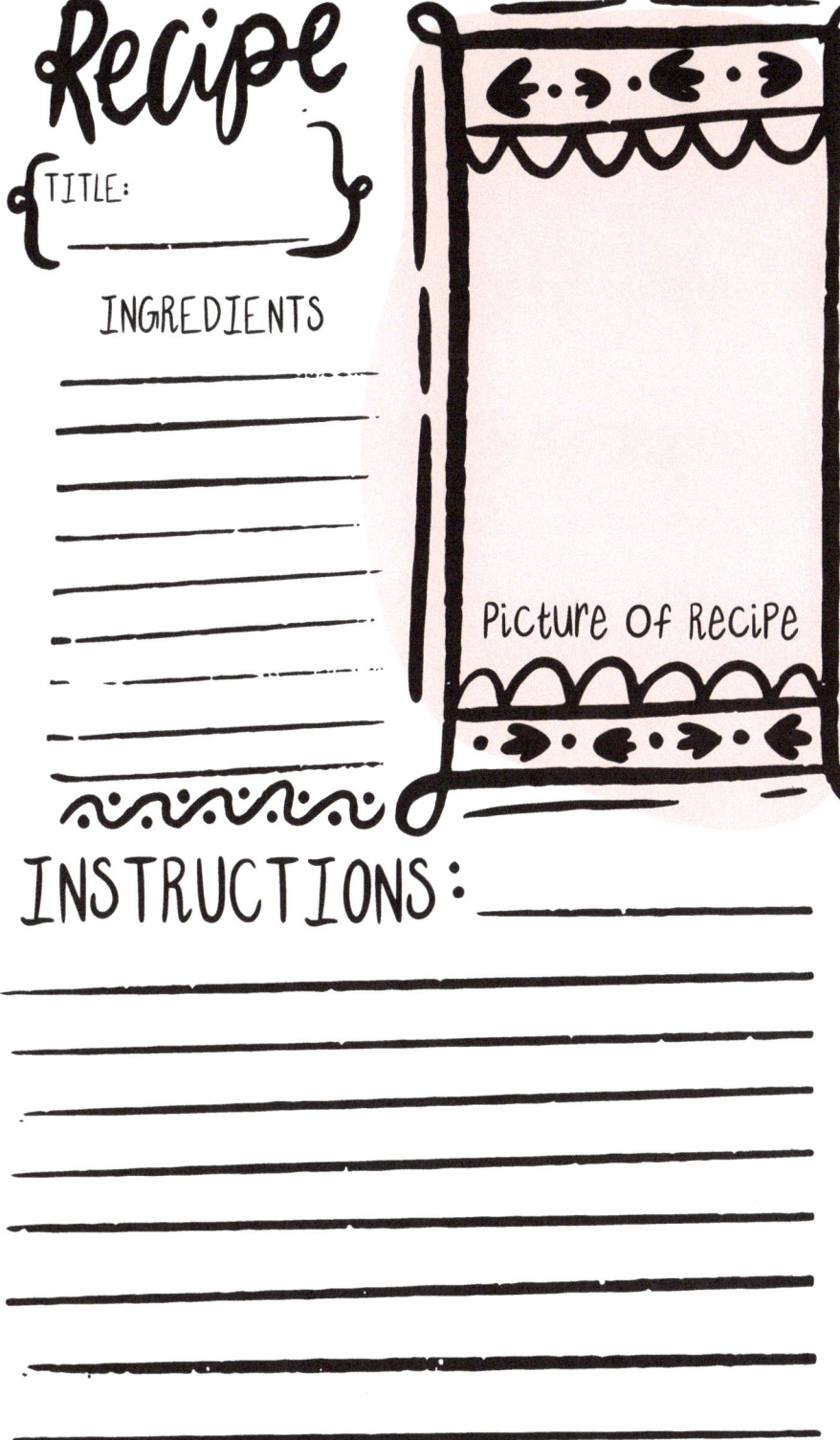

Picture Of Recipe

INSTRUCTIONS: _____

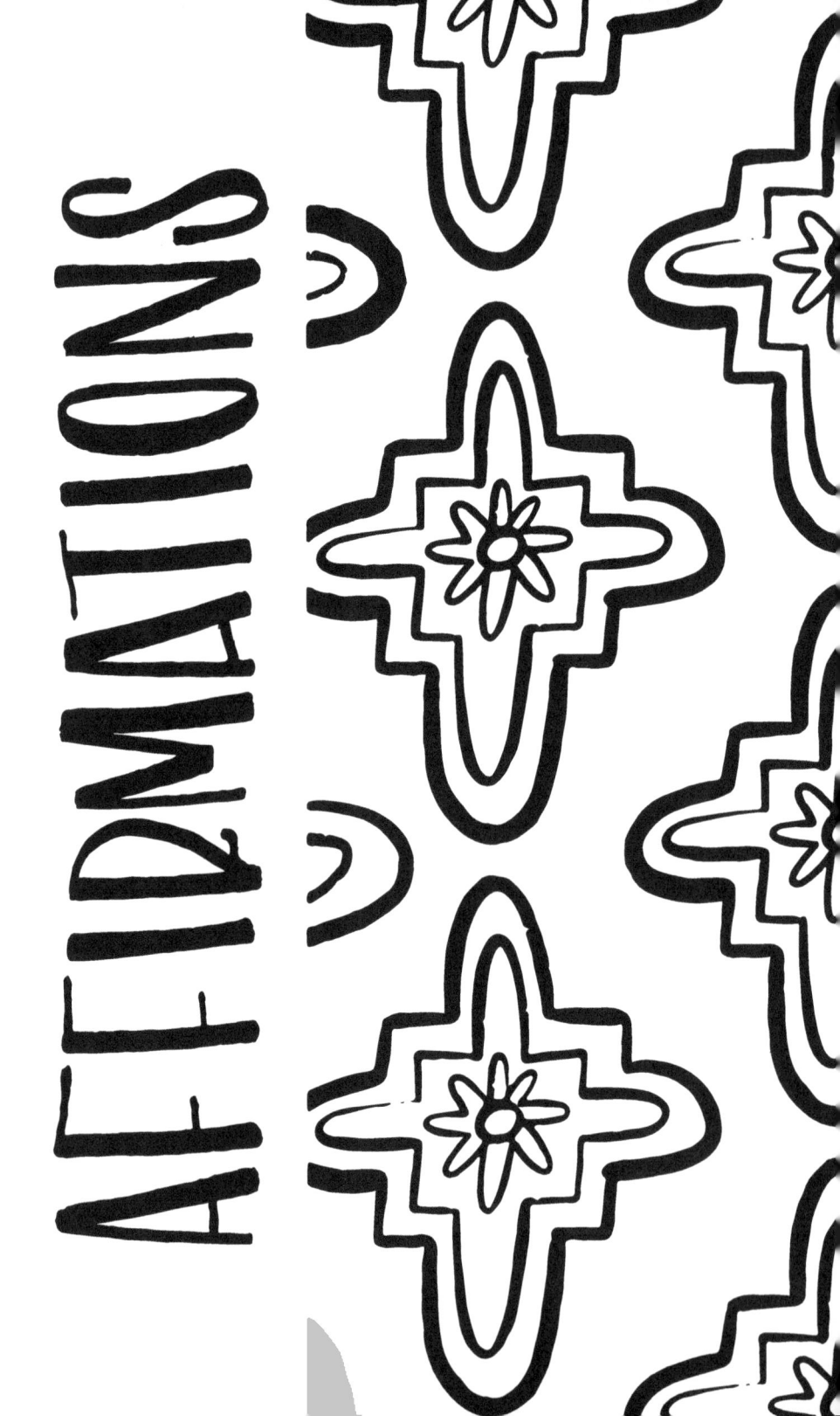

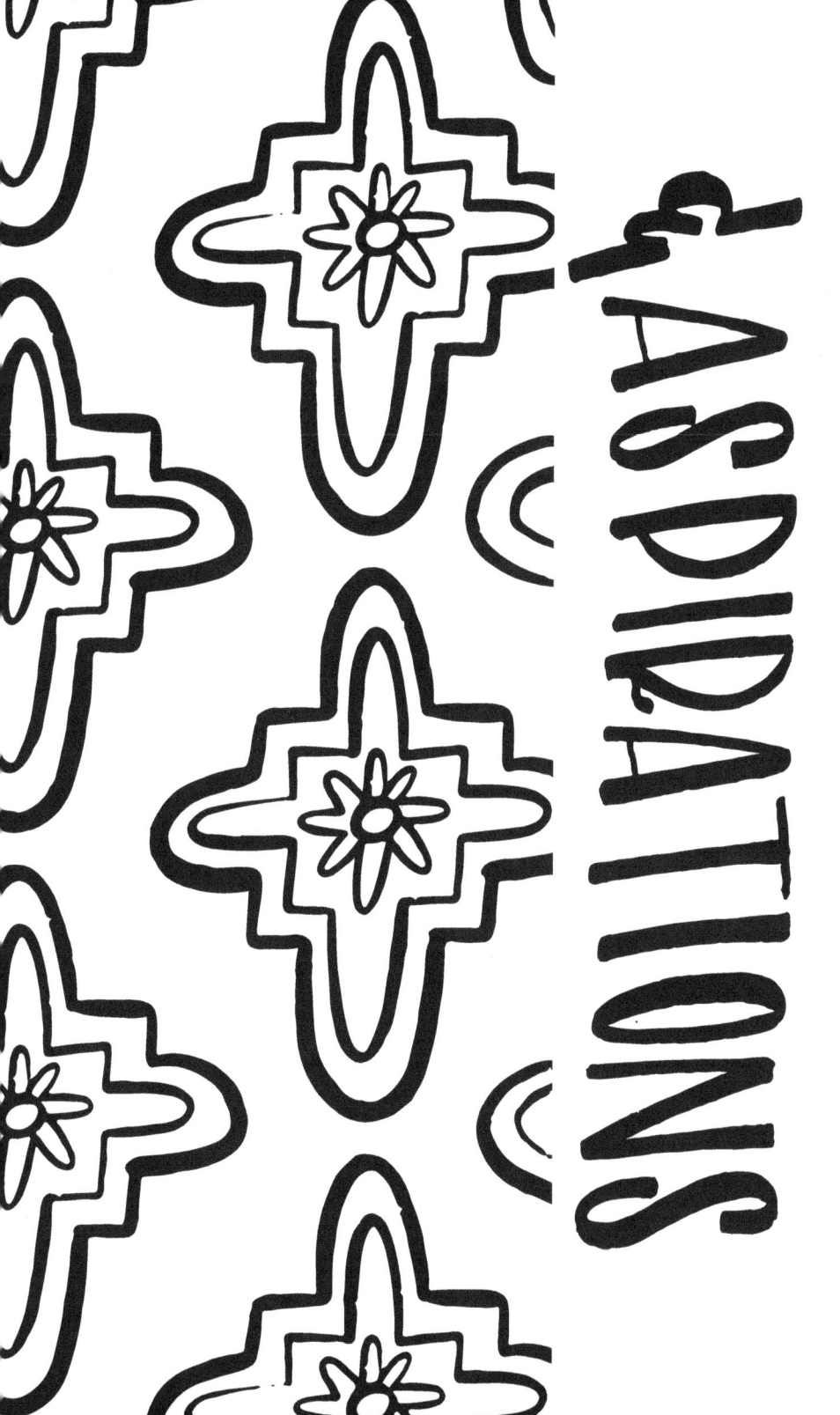

goals & intentions

RELATIONSHIP	HEALTH
PERSONAL	**CAREER**
FINANCE	**SPIRITUAL**

GOALS ACHIEVED	WANT TO ACHIEVE

SUMMARIES YOUR DREAMS

1
_____
_____
_____
_____
_____

2
_____
_____
_____
_____
_____

3
_____
_____
_____
_____
_____

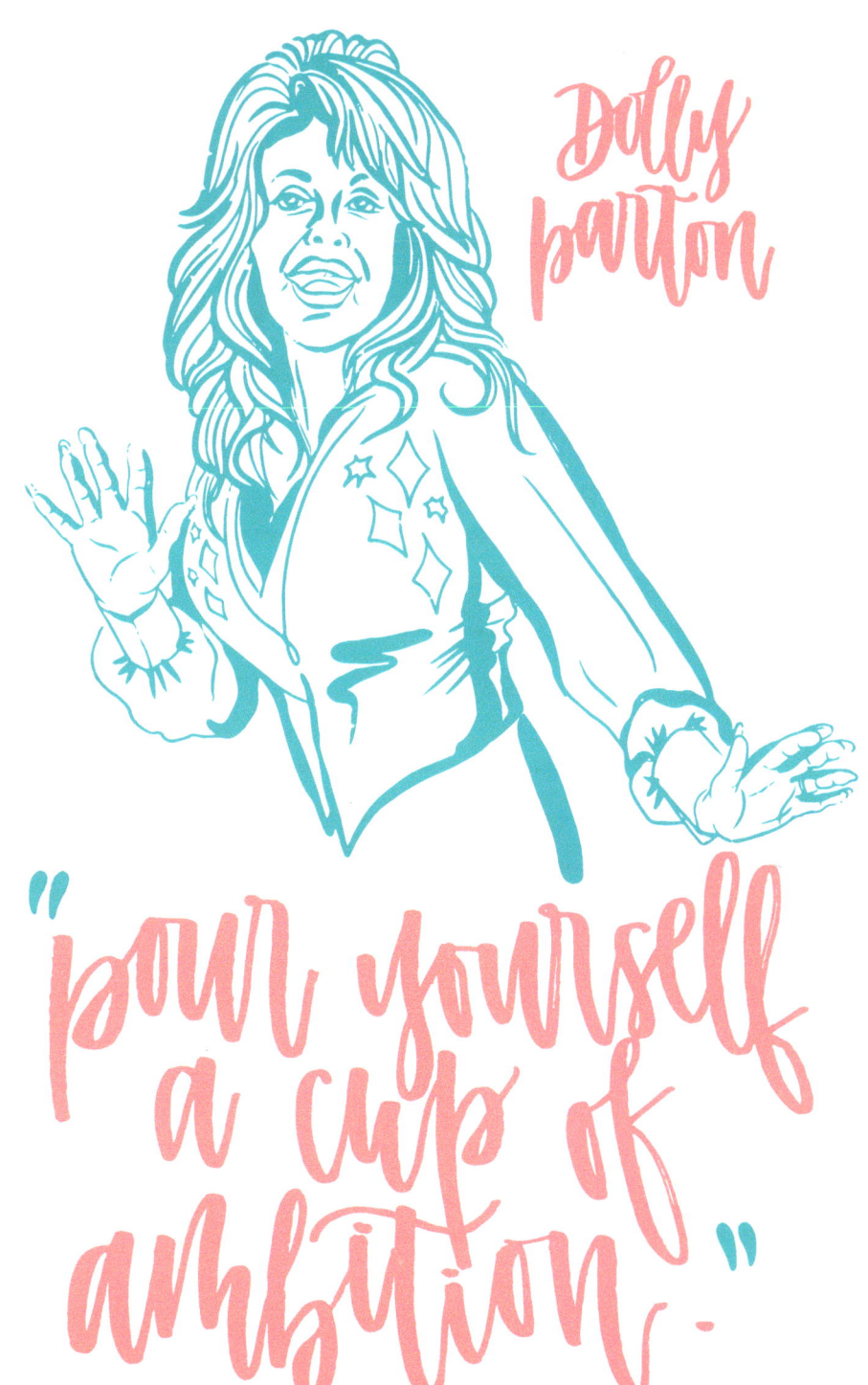

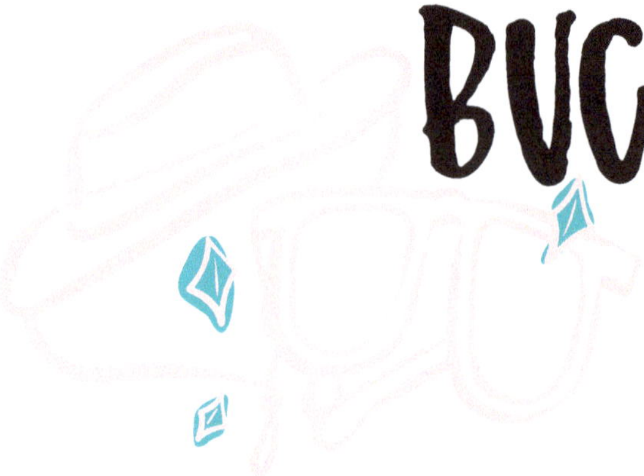

BUCKET LIST

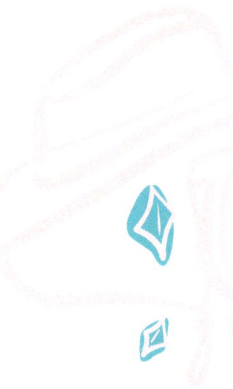

What is on your Bucket List and Why?

1. _____
   _____
   _____

2. _____
   _____
   _____

3. _____
   _____
   _____

4. _____
   _____
   _____

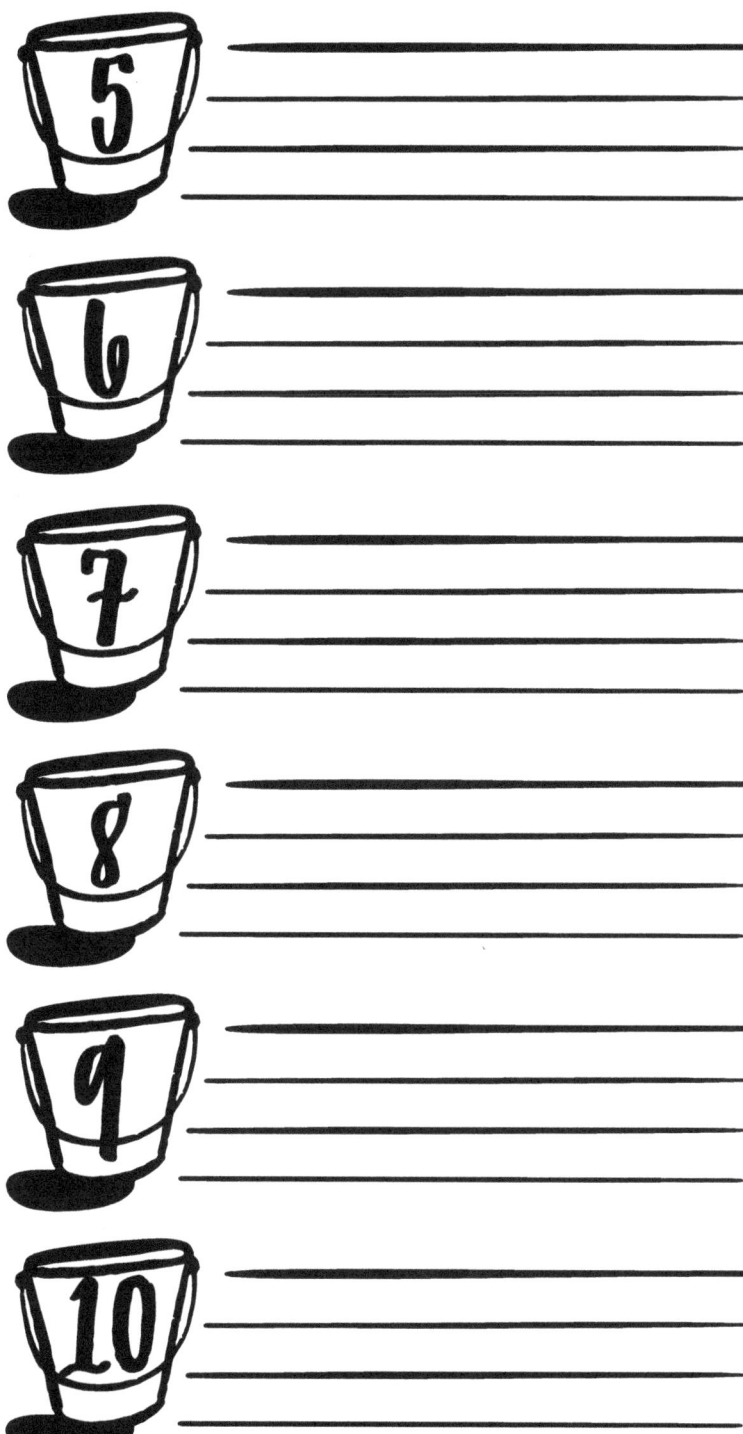

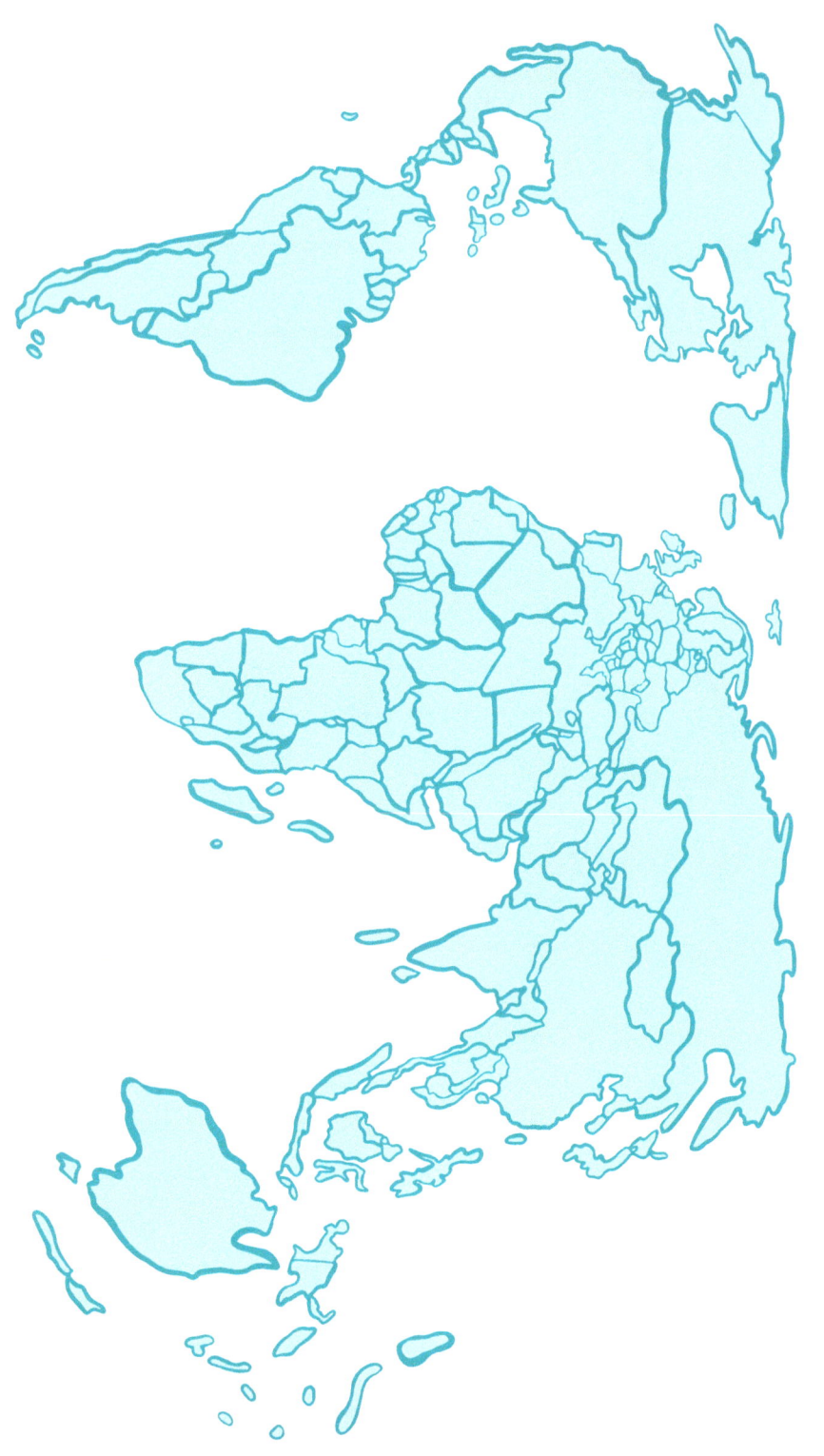

top 5 destinations
(where & why)

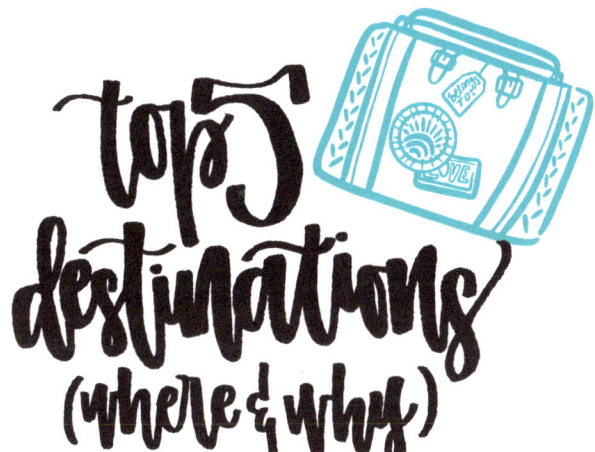

1. _____

2. _____

3. _____

4. _____

5. _____

SET A SAVINGS GOAL AND SHADE AS YOU SAVE!

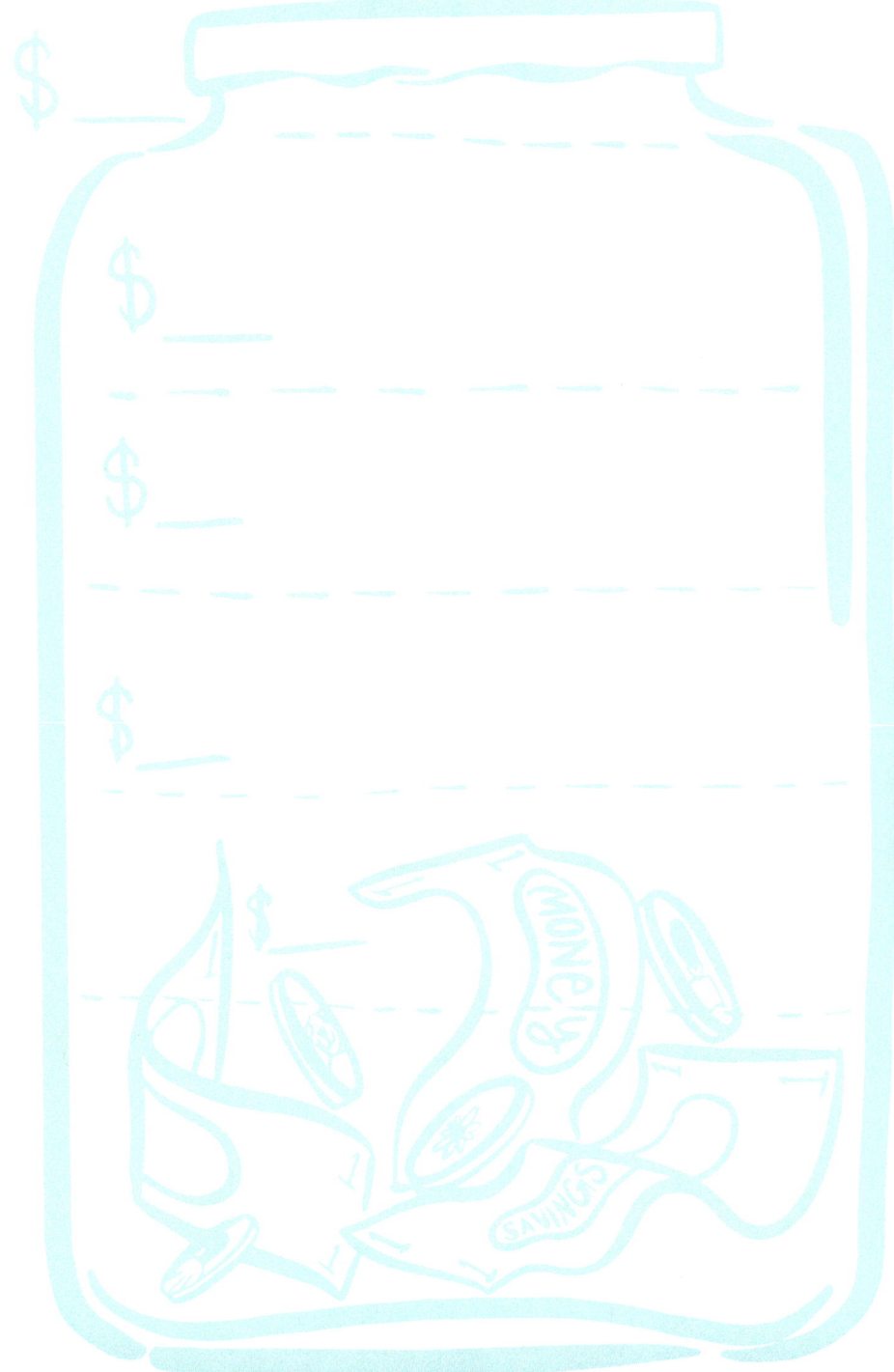

"The key to realizing a dream is to focus not on success but on significance - and then even the small steps and little victories along your path will take on greater meaning."

-Oprah Winfrey

What are you Grateful for?

Where do you see yourself in five years?

What do you love about yourself?

what are ways to gain confidence?

What can you do to make someone smile?

What is one thing about yourself you're proud of?

What defines success?

What are your favorite things?

what memories bring you joy?

Who is your favorite person? Why?

What are your values?

What can you tell yourself to motivate positivity?

Best things to do on a rainy day?

who are you thankful for?

What's you're dream vacation?

If you were famous, what would be your talent?

words of wisdom from your elders?

what makes your soul smile?

How can you give more to others in life?

What's the best lesson you've ever learned?

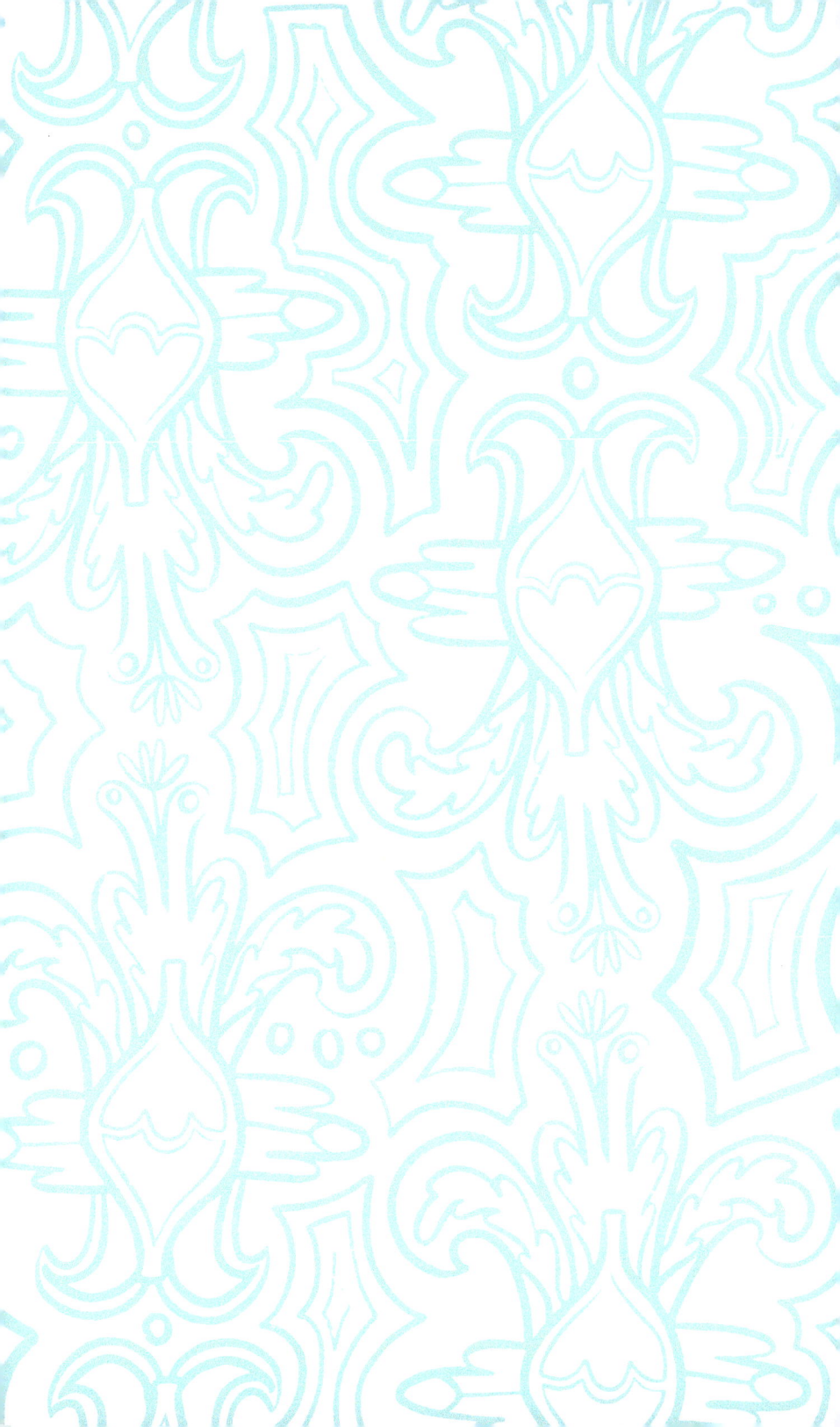

SHE NEEDED A HERO. SO THAT'S WHAT SHE BECAME.

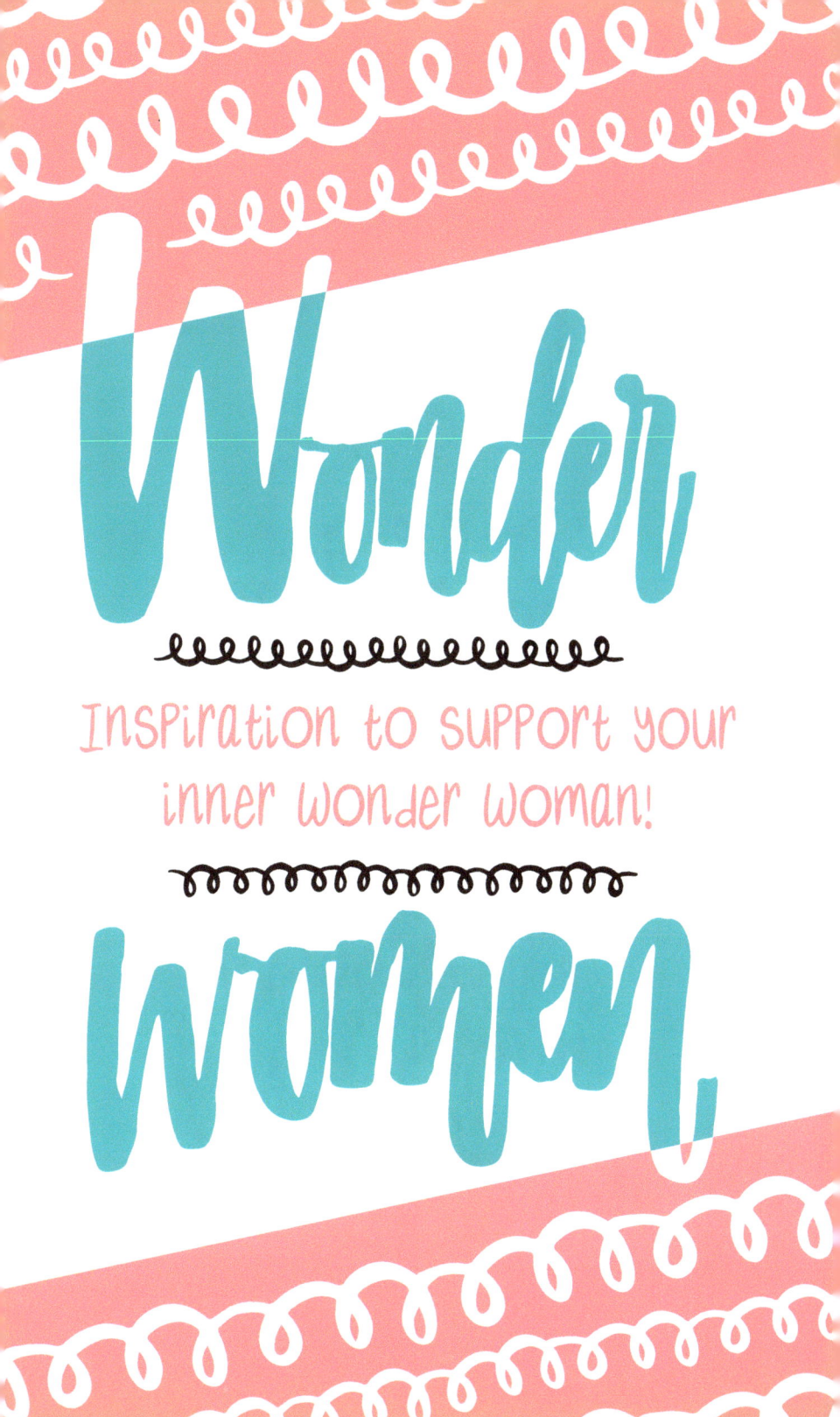

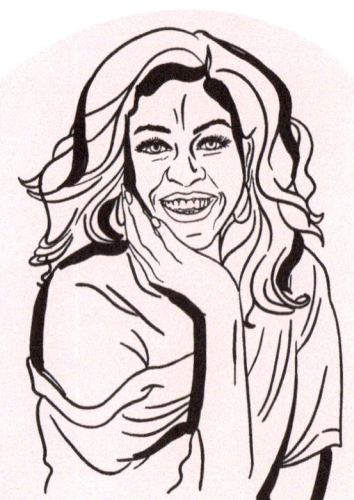

"Don't ever underestimate the importance you can have because history has shown us that courage can be contagious & hope can take on a life of its own."

michelle obama

"Other women who are killing it should motivate you, thrill you, challenge you, & inspire you." — Taylor Swift

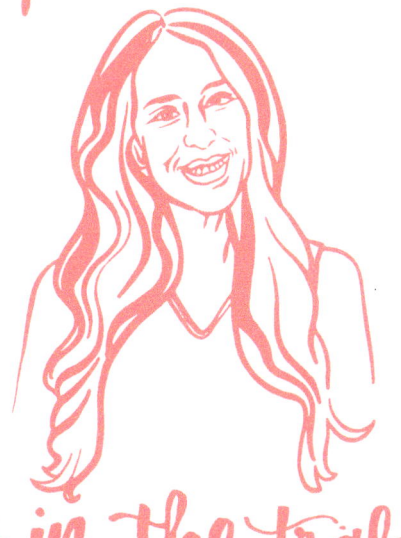

"Even in the trials of life, if we have eyes to see them, we can find good things everywhere we look."

Joanna Gaines

self reflection

"Challenges are gifts that force us to search for a new center of gravity. Don't fight them. Just find a new way to stand."

—Oprah

"Life is not measured by the number of breaths we take, but by the moments that take our breath away."

MAYA ANGELOU

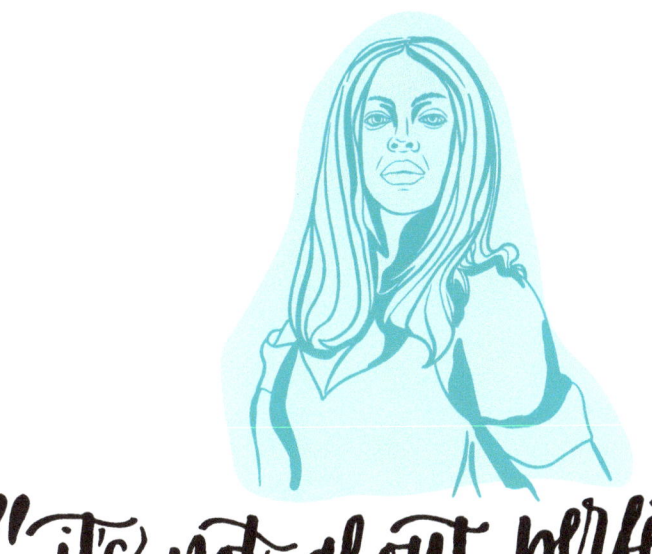

"It's not about perfection. It's about purpose." BEYONCÉ

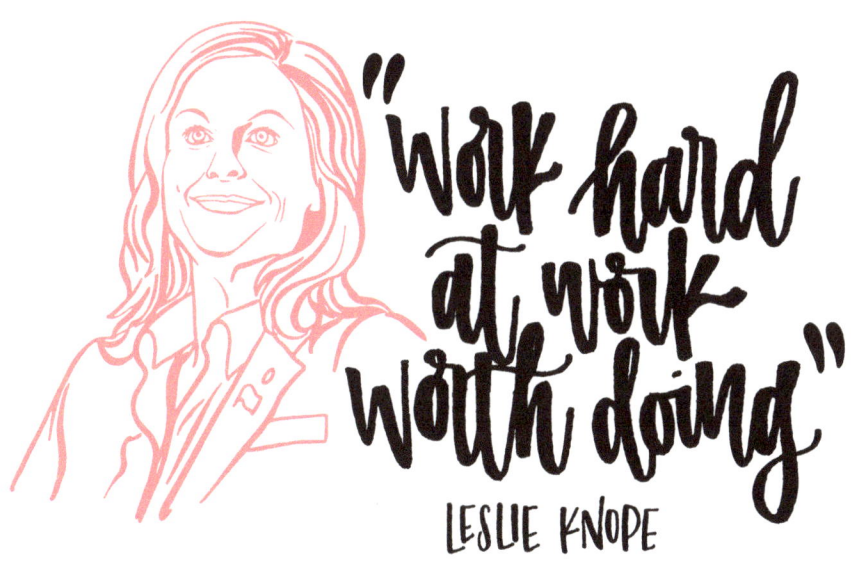

"Work hard at work worth doing"
LESLIE KNOPE

"To be liberated women must feel free to be herself, not in rivalry to man but in the context of her own capacity and her personality."

INDIRA GANDHI

What inspires me?

___

How can I inspire others?

___

MOTIVATIONAL QUOTES FROM LOCAL QUEENS

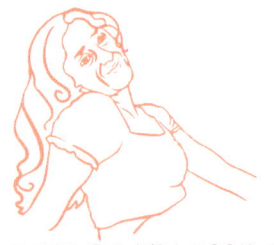
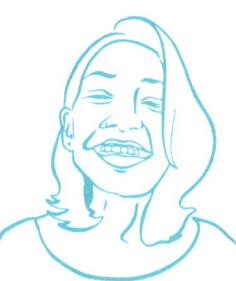

"HARD WORK DOES PAY OFF EVENTUALLY. KEEP HUSTLING!"
AIMEE JONES

"WE'RE TOO BUSY CARING ABOUT BECOMING BETTER WHEN YOU'RE ALREADY THE PERSON YOUR YOUNGER SELF WANTED TO BE!"
MEGHNA KINSHORE

"WE'RE TESTED BECAUSE WE CAN MAKE IT TO THE END"
GEETIKA GAUTAM

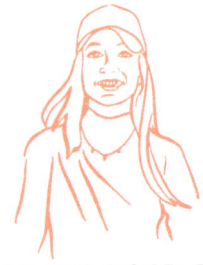
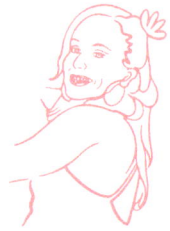

"THE MOST IMPORTANT COMMITMENT THAT YOU'LL EVER MAKE IS TO WRITING YOUR OWN STORY IN A WAY THAT WILL BENEFIT THE WHOLE WORLD."
DENISA MENTEA

"YOU HAVE TO CHOOSE TO LOVE YOURSELF BEFORE YOU CAN LEARN TO LOVE OTHERS FULLY."
SAVANNAH KARAS

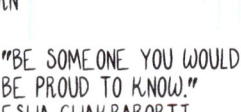

"BE SOMEONE YOU WOULD BE PROUD TO KNOW."
ESHA CHAKRABORTI

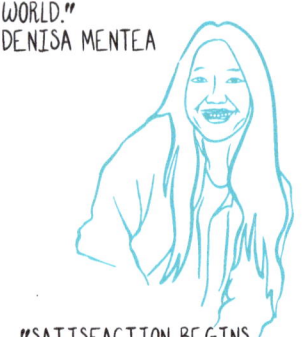
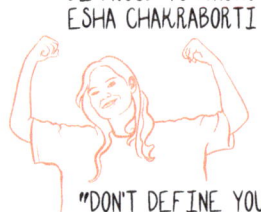

"DON'T DEFINE YOURSELF BY OTHERS CRITISISM."
ELIZABETH COX

"SATISFACTION BEGINS WHERE EXPECTATIONS END"
TONYA HU

"DON'T BE DISCOURAGED WHEN YOU'RE ON A DIFFICULT ROAD NOBODY ELSE IS ON. MAYBE YOU'RE MEANT TO SEE SOMETHING THAT CHANGES YOUR VISION OF THE WORLD. THE MOST BEAUTIFUL PLACES ON EARTH ARE USUALLY THE MOST HIDDEN FROM PEOPLE."
HELEN KALLEB

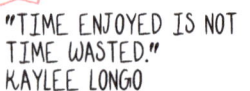
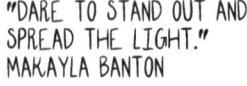

"TIME ENJOYED IS NOT TIME WASTED."
KAYLEE LONGO

"DARE TO STAND OUT AND SPREAD THE LIGHT."
MAKAYLA BANTON

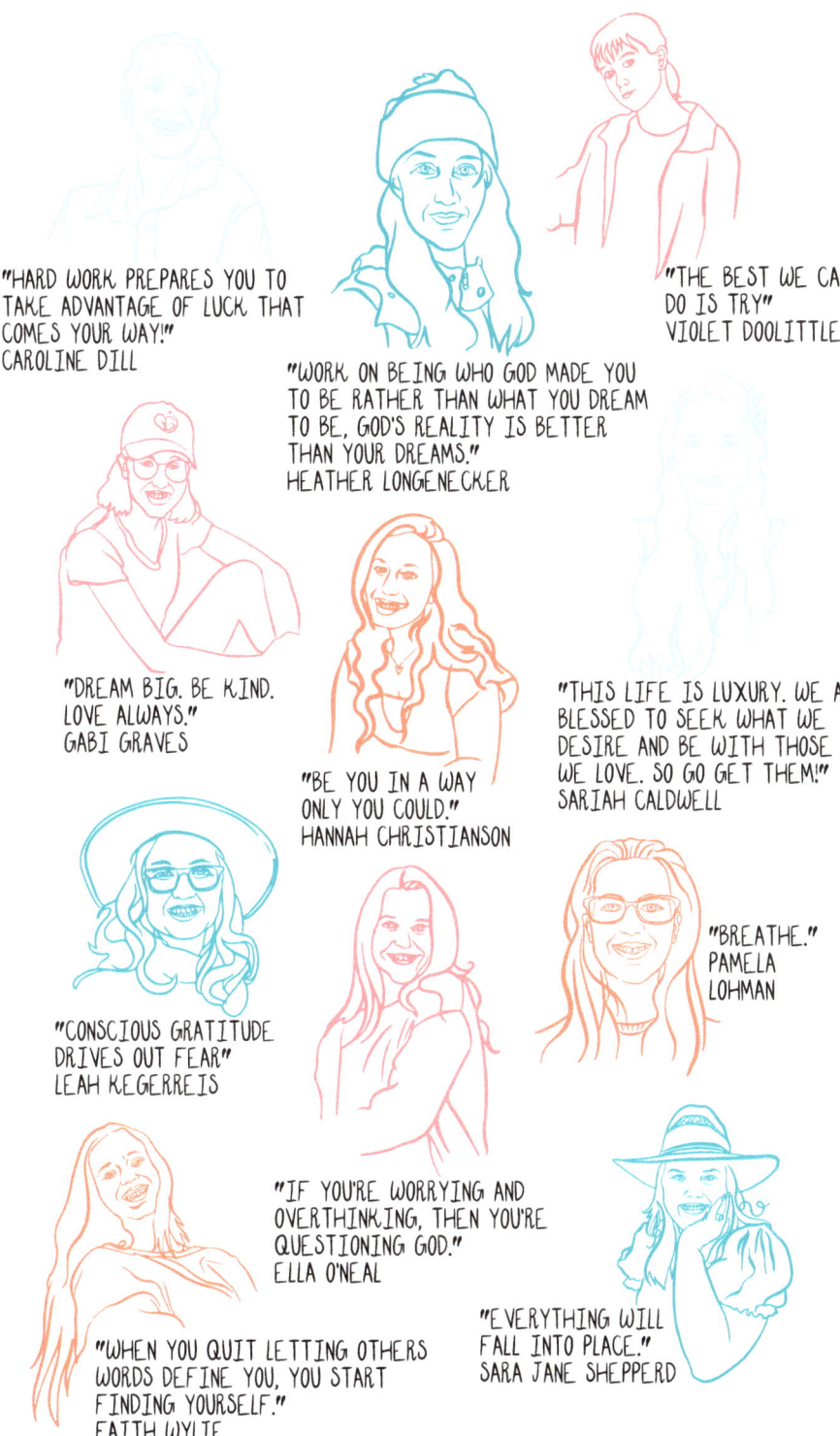

my mantra

WHAT UNIQUE WORDS OF MOTIVATIONAL WISDOM WOULD YOU LIKE TO SHARE WITH THE WORLD?

_____

_____

_____

_____

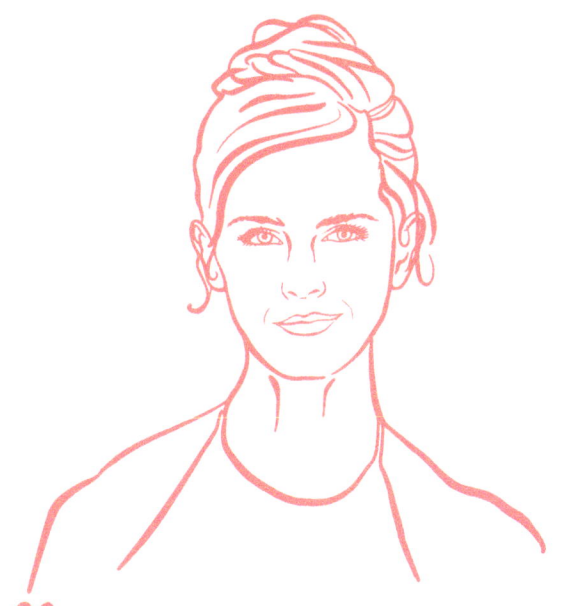

The end is just the Beginning

CONGRATULATIONS ON REACHING THE END OF THE BOOK! WE HOPE THIS HAS SPARKED SOME INSPIRATION, JOY, AND GOOD JUJU TO TAKE INTO YOUR LIFE EVERY SINGLE DAY! YOU ARE SO BEAUTIFULLY AND WONDERFULLY MADE, SO GO INTO YOUR LIFE WITH A SMILE ON YOUR FACE. YOU ARE GOING TO HAVE BAD DAYS, BAD WEEKS, BAD MONTHS, BUT IF YOU LOOK FOR THE GOOD IN THE PRESENT MOMENT, FOR WE ASSURE YOU THERE IS GOOD, YOU WILL FIND GRATITUDE IN THE PERSON STARING BACK IN THE MIRROR. WE ARE ALL FAR FROM PERFECT, WE ARE ARTISTS IN OUR OWN MANNER CAPTURING MEMORIES AND THOUGHTS WHILE TRANSFORMING THEM INTO OUR DREAMS AND REALITIES. DON'T LET ANYONE TELL YOU YOU ARE NOT WORTH IT, YOU CAN'T DO IT, YOU'RE NOT STRONG ENOUGH BECAUSE YOU ARE. THROUGH AND THROUGH. THERE'S A WORLD AWAITING YOUR PRESENCE AND YOU MAY NEVER FIND THE PERFECT PATH, BUT HAVE CONFIDENCE IN THAT. HAVE CONFIDENCE IN YOUR
JOURNEY, EXPLORE AND BE CURIOUS, FOR THERE IS NO MOMENT LIKE THE PRESENT TO BECOME THE BEST YOU THAT YOU CAN BE!
LOVE,
MEL AND MADDIE

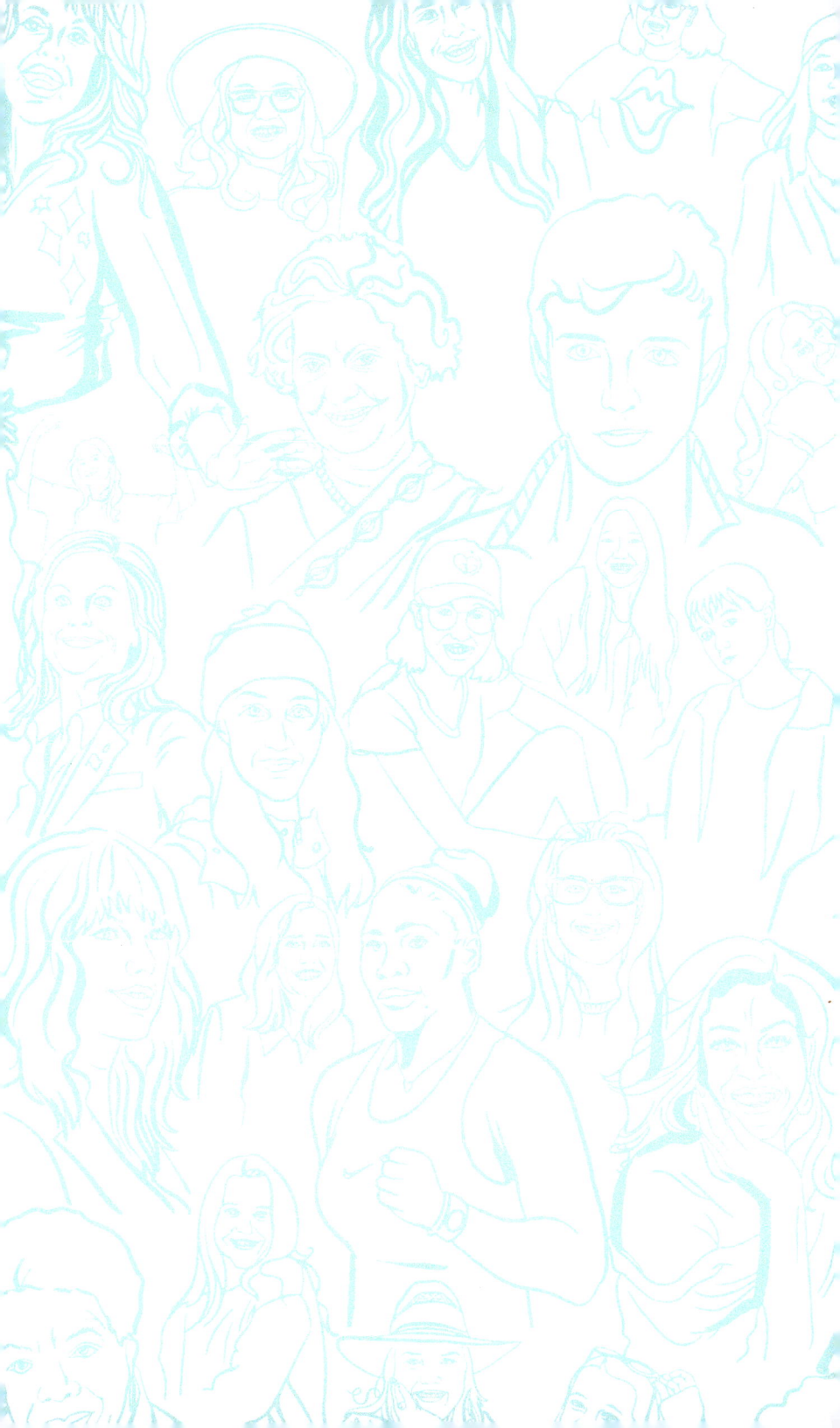

THANK YOU

CPSIA information can be obtained
at www.ICGtesting.com
Printed in the USA
BVHW060514150821
614412BV00003B/18